PROXIMAL FEMORAL FOCAL DEFICIENCY
A Congenital Anomaly

A SYMPOSIUM
Held in Washington, D.C.
June 13, 1968

Subcommittee on Child Prosthetics Problems
Committee on Prosthetics Research and Development
Division of Engineering
of the
National Research Council

NATIONAL ACADEMY OF SCIENCES
Washington, D.C.   1969

Standard Book Number 309-01734-3

Available from

Printing and Publishing Office
National Academy of Sciences
2101 Constitution Avenue
Washington, D.C. 20418

Library of Congress Catalog Card No.: 73-602074

Foreword

The papers in this monograph were presented at the 1968 Annual Clinic Chiefs' Meeting, sponsored by the Subcommittee on Child Prosthetics Problems of the Committee on Prosthetics Research and Development of the National Research Council. The members of the symposium were orthopedic surgeons, prosthetists, and allied personnel with a rich background of experience and expertness in treating the complex deformity, proximal femoral deficiency.

As these papers make clear, there is a great deal of interest and controversy concerning the surgical procedures and management of patients with anomalies of the proximal femur. One, or both, lower extremities may be affected in varying degrees. When both are involved, the problem is usually more severe. One of the major difficulties is the extreme loss of height. There is no simple approach to treatment which can be applied to every patient. Each child's condition requires individual analysis. The decision as to the direction and timing of the child's treatment program involves both surgical and prosthetics judgment, as well as discussion of the problem with the parents and with the child, if he is old enough to participate.

This monograph brings together the best that is known regarding the adequate classification of the types of abnormalities that are encountered and the therapeutic techniques required in the treatment of these limb-deprived children.

The Children's Bureau is pleased to have had a part in sponsoring this symposium.

Arthur J. Lesser, M.D.

Preface

In planning the scientific portion of the program, represented by the papers which comprise this volume, the existence of a great deal of controversy concerning the management of patients with a partial or complete absence of the proximal femur was recognized. Moreover, as interest in the combined surgical and prosthetic management of limb-deficient children has increased, it has become apparent that anomalies of the proximal femur present a major problem.

The literature contains many isolated case reports but only a few papers of any depth. Prior to this meeting, detailed discussions with adequate numbers of cases and length of follow-up to substantiate claims for proposed therapy techniques were nonexistent.

The mature clinician is aware of the paucity of specifics in both medicine and surgery. Treatment in general represents the establishment of a diagnosis, a knowledge of the life history of the disease or anomaly, and then the judicious application of medical or surgical principles, varied as necessary for the individual patient involved.

What has been lacking for some time in the problem of proximal femoral deficiencies has been an adequate classification of the varieties of abnormalities encountered and a sufficient understanding of their natural life history. Their etiology is as yet undetermined. Their contribution to functional loss, however, is recognized and can be categorized.

Principles of reconstructive surgery about the hip have been established. Mobility, stability, and freedom from pain are well-known criteria. To attain them all is the ideal desideratum. To know when to attain one at the expense of the others is to have impeccable judgment.

In this confusing group of cases the diagnosis and establishment of a long-term treatment program is often difficult, particularly for the young clinician.

This symposium was developed around a group of surgeons who had developed expertise in this problem and whose clinical situations had permitted them to see instances of the anomaly in larger volume than is usual.

Since classification and knowledge of the anomaly's natural life history seem of fundamental importance, there has been emphasis on these aspects of the problem. Dr. Aitken's classification of the proximal femoral deficiency is based on a survey of thirty-five cases, many of them observed through skeletal maturity. This series permits classification and establishes the natural life history of the deficiency. Dr. Amstutz modifies this plan to include a classification of the total femoral involvement, and he also develops a concept of prediction of final leg-length inequality.

These approaches are not incompatible and, whether combined or used in isolation, they establish a diagnosis. On the basis of a predictable life history, treatment plans can be more accurately developed. These papers present a model for analysis of the biomechanical loss. This approach tends to pinpoint the areas in which treatment is needed. Finally, there are sufficient follow-up and carefully observed functional results to make it possible to assess the functional gain afforded by various types of treatment.

Dr. King's paper focuses mainly on indications for the need to promote increased stability at the hip with retention of adequate mobility and painlessness, and on the methods used to achieve this stability.

The paper of Dr. Hall and Mr. Bochmann is concerned primarily with the presentation of their experiences with the Van Nes procedure. This peripheral reconstruction procedure permits fitting with a below-knee type of prosthesis under active muscular control. With or without proximal reconstruction, there are good theoretical reasons for conversion to a below-knee rather than an above-knee type.

The paper of Drs. Westin and Gunderson provides a careful summary of the results of various therapeutic approaches to this problem by surgeons in different areas of the country. It is an honest, retrospective analysis of results and deserves very careful study.

The Subcommittee on Child Prosthetics Problems hopes that a careful review of these papers will establish a sound, in-depth picture of proximal femoral deficiencies. Classifications of prosthetic applications possible and indications for the use of each, with and without supplemental surgical reconstruction of the anomaly, are also dealt with in detail.

The differences in opinion that become evident with careful reading should enhance the value of the monograph in that they emphasize the fact that there is no single best way to classify and manage all cases.

In a high percentage of cases, this anomaly is associated with other skeletal deficiencies in the same and other limbs. Most such patients are, therefore, "multihandicapped" and so have a more limited rehabilitation potential than the child with a single limb deficiency. All clinicians responsible for the establishment of a treatment program for such patients must be very certain that, on the basis of documented experience, their plan for treatment will produce improved function. These already severely handicapped patients can ill afford an iatrogenic increase in functional loss.

Organization of the symposium and publication of this report were part of the work conducted under a grant to the National Academy of Sciences–National Research Council from the Children's Bureau, Department of Health, Education, and Welfare.

The assistance of Hector W. Kay, Enid N. Partin, and Milda H. Vaivada in the preparation of this publication is gratefully acknowledged.

GEORGE T. AITKEN, M.D., *Chairman*
Subcommittee on Child Prosthetics Problems

Subcommittee on Child Prosthetics Problems

COMMITTEE ON PROSTHETICS RESEARCH AND DEVELOPMENT
DIVISION OF ENGINEERING
NATIONAL RESEARCH COUNCIL
NATIONAL ACADEMY OF SCIENCES-NATIONAL ACADEMY OF ENGINEERING

George T. Aitken, M.D., *Chairman*

Sidney Fishman, Ph.D.

Claude N. Lambert, M.D.

Fred Leonard, Ph.D.

Colin A. McLaurin

Yoshio Setoguchi, M.D.

Contents

GEORGE T. AITKEN, M.D.

PROXIMAL FEMORAL FOCAL DEFICIENCY–
Definition, Classification, and Management

Congenital anomalies of the proximal femur with or without involvement of the iliofemoral joint have been observed and reported for many years (1). The condition that has probably been best described and documented is congenital or infantile coxa vara (3-5, 7, 9, 12).

As interest increased in the prosthetic treatment of certain skeletal limb deficiencies, the existence of a group of partial deficiencies of the proximal femur involving the iliofemoral joint became evident. These conditions were poorly documented and unclassified. Neither the Frantz-O'Rahilly (6) nor the Hall (10) classification system for skeletal limb deficiencies, for example, provides terminology for partial absence of either the femur or the humerus. Hence, the designation "proximal femoral focal deficiency," or PFFD, was coined for this group of cases. This paper presents the clinical and radiologic life history of this condition and outlines the author's experiences and recommendations for treatment.

The clinical experience with this anomaly at the Area Child Amputee Center in Grand Rapids, Michigan, may be summarized as follows: Of 35 cases considered to January 1, 1968, there were 21 males and 14 females; of these 35 cases, 11 had right involvement, 19 left, and 5 bilateral. The typical clinical picture is clearly shown in Figure 1. In severe cases, diagnosis can be made by inspection. On the affected side there is a short femoral segment that is flexed, abducted, and externally rotated. The tibia may or may not be of normal length. Usually the sole of the foot on the affected side is about at the level of the contralateral knee joint.

When serial x-rays of these patients are reviewed over a considerable period of time, it is possible to identify four radiologic subclasses of this condition (2). Figure 2 shows an artist's representation of the four radiologic subclasses.

SUBCLASSES

In Class A a head of the femur is present, together with an adequate acetabulum and a very short femoral segment. Initially, there is no bony connection between the segment and the head of the femur. At skeletal maturity in this subtype a bony connection is present between the shaft of the femur and the head, neck, and trochanteric component. In most instances a pseudarthrosis is evident at their point of connection, and this defect does not heal in all instances. It is possible that for this class the term PFFD is semantically incorrect because basically there is no deficiency in the proximal femur at skeletal maturity. There is simply inequality of femoral lengths and an abnormal relationship between the head, neck, and trochanteric component of the femur and its shaft, with severe subtrochanteric varus. This group is included in PFFD because the clinical picture is essentially identical with that of the other three groups.

The characteristics of Class B are the presence of a head of the femur and an adequate acetabulum, together with a short, deformed femoral shaft, usually with a small bony tuft on its proximal end. At skeletal maturity there is no osseous connection between the femoral head and shaft. Cineradiographic studies done on these children at skeletal maturity demonstrate that the head does not move synchronously with motions of the shaft of the femur, and, therefore, it is believed that there is no cartilaginous connection between the shaft and head and neck segments.

In Class C the acetabulum is severely dysplastic. The head of the femur never ossifies and it is believed that there is no cartilaginous model of the femoral head. The shaft of the femur is short with an ossified tuft at the proximal end of the shaft.

Class D is characterized by the absence of both the

1

acetabulum and femoral head; by a deformed, shortened femoral shaft; and by no proximal tufting on the shaft of the femur.

It is important to recognize that although the clinical picture seems to be identical in all of these cases, review of x-rays throughout the period of a patient's pre- and post-skeletal maturity demonstrates the presence of four radiologic subclassifications. Further discussion of these types, with a presentation of illustrative cases, follows.

CLASS A PROXIMAL FEMORAL FOCAL DEFICIENCY

An example of Class A PFFD is shown in Figure 3-A. This child's heel is about level with the contralateral knee joint. The shaft of the femur is very short, and there is associated fibular hemimelia. The flexion, abduction, and external rotation deformities in this hip are not as characteristically extensive as those found in most of these patients.

The radiograph in Figure 3-B was taken when the patient was one day old. No acetabulum is evident and the shaft of the femur is very short. The femur rides laterally in relationship to the ilium. The associated fibular hemimelia on the same side can be observed.

At six years of age (Figure 3-C) the head of the femur is ossified. The shaft of the femur is now riding above the acetabulum. A distal femoral epiphysis is evident, together with an amorphous calcification of what is probably a cartilaginous anlage of the greater and lesser trochanters and the base of the femoral neck.

An x-ray of the same patient at twelve years and four months is shown in Figure 3-D. The head, neck, and greater and lesser trochanters are now ossified, but there is a pseudarthrosis between these components and the shaft. A severe varus deformity is evident. It should be emphasized that this is a subtrochanteric varus and is not a neck–shaft varus as is seen in typical infantile coxa vara. It is this appearance that oftentimes leads observers to mistakenly confuse Class A PFFD with congenital or infantile coxa vara. Careful review of x-rays, such as those in Figure 3-D, in comparison with those of typical infantile coxa vara, will demonstrate the difference in the location of the varus deformity and will also demonstrate that the defect in the PFFD is subtrochanteric, whereas the defect in infantile coxa vara is at the level of the subcapital epiphysis.

At twenty years of age, ossification of the head, neck, and trochanters has progressed (Figure 3-E), but a pseudarthrosis between the head, neck, and trochanteric segments and the shaft persists. A severe, persistent subtrochanteric varus is also present.

CLASS B PROXIMAL FEMORAL FOCAL DEFICIENCY

A representative clinical example of Class B is shown in Figure 4-A. On the affected side there is a very short femoral segment, a short tibial segment, and a deformed foot that extends to about the level of the opposite knee joint. The child has numerous other limb deficiencies.

X-rays of this patient at eleven months of age (Figure 4-B) demonstrate that, although an acetabulum is evident, the femoral head has not yet ossified, and the shaft of the femur is short, flexed, abducted, and externally rotated. An associated fibular hemimelia is apparent on the same side.

The status of the same patient at ten years and nine months is shown in Figure 4-C. It is now evident that there is a head in the acetabulum and that the head is ossified. The shaft of the femur still rides high, and at the proximal end of the femoral shaft there appears to be a calcific tuft which may represent a trochanteric apophysis. Cineradiographic studies in this case demonstrate that there is no synchronous motion of the head with the shaft. This evidence tends to substantiate the concept that there is no cartilaginous connection between the femoral shaft and the ossified head of the femur.

CLASS C PROXIMAL FEMORAL FOCAL DEFICIENCY

Figure 5-A presents the characteristic clinical picture of Class C PFFD. An x-ray of this patient at age two months (Figure 5-B) shows the very short shaft of the femur, a moderately inadequate acetabulum, and fibular hemimelia on the same side. The total leg length on the affected side is essentially equal to the femoral segment on the contralateral side.

X-rays of the patient at eleven years and eleven months of age are shown in Figure 5-C. The dysplasia of the acetabulum can be noted. There is no ossification of the head of the femur on that side, and the shaft of the femur rides proximal and posterior to the ilium.

CLASS D PROXIMAL FEMORAL FOCAL DEFICIENCY

The patient shown in Figure 6-A is a bilateral PFFD, Class D. An x-ray of this patient at the age of seven years and five months is shown in Figure 6-B. Attention is directed to the obliquity of the lateral walls of the pelvis. No ossification of the femoral heads has occurred and no acetabula are present. The femora are very short and are flexed, abducted, and externally rotated. No proximal tufts of ossification are evident on the femora.

X-rays of the same patient at eleven years and five months of age are shown in Figure 6-C.

DIFFERENTIAL DIAGNOSES

The differential diagnosis of this condition is generally not difficult. Figure 7-A demonstrates a patient with a very short femoral segment, some flexion, some abduction and external rotation, and marked inequality of leg lengths. X-rays of this patient taken at one month (Figure 7-B) show that she has a very short femoral segment, does have an acetabulum, and the femur is laterally displaced with marked shortening as compared to the opposite side. It is possible to confuse this condition with either a Class A or a Class B PFFD at this age. Radiographs at age eight years and four months (Figure 7-C) demonstrate that this patient does have infantile coxa vara. This is a neck–shaft varus, with deformation of all of the components of the head, neck, and trochanteric area, and shortening of the femur. This condition represents idiopathic or juvenile or congenital coxa vara associated with congenital shortening of the femur (*8*). This is an entirely different entity, and the differential diagnosis between congenital coxa vara with a short femur and PFFD Class A or B is generally best made by x-ray at approximately one year of age.

The x-rays of a three-day-old patient (Figure 8-A) illustrate another possible problem of differential diagnosis. This patient does have an acetabulum, a short femur, and an anterolateral bowing of the femur in its midshaft. X-rays of this child at fifteen months (Figure 8-B) demonstrate an adequate acetabulum, a quite normal femoral head, proximal epiphysis, neck, greater and lesser trochanters, and a quite normal femoral shaft except that it is short and the antero-lateral bowing at its midportion is gradually clearing. It is interesting to note that this patient has an incomplete fibular hemimelia on the same side. Figure 8-B demonstrates the shortening of the fibula on the affected as compared to the unaffected side. This patient does have leg-length inequality because of both femoral and tibial shortening. At the present time there is no established classification for this combination of congenital skeletal limb deficiencies. Patients with this condition may often be confused with PFFD Class A or B at birth, but by six months of age the x-rays clearly differentiate these two conditions.

TREATMENT

Patients with proximal femoral focal deficiency, either unilateral or bilateral, have a relatively high incidence of associated skeletal limb deficiencies. For instance, in a study of 29 cases, 68.9 percent had fibular hemimelia in the same limb, and 51.7 percent had other skeletal deficiencies in other limbs. From these figures it seems evident that in many instances patients with PFFD fall into the category of the multihandicapped child.

The biomechanical losses in children with lower-extremity skeletal limb deficiencies can be characterized as:

1. Inequality of leg length
2. Malrotation
3. Inadequacy of proximal musculature
4. Instability of proximal joints

Patients with proximal femoral focal deficiency exhibit most of these characteristics. They have inequality of leg lengths; there is malrotation of the limb; there is inadequacy of proximal joints; and the proximal musculature is also inadequate.

The concept of treating these children prosthetically is based on the fact that prosthetic application will correct or at least improve many of the biomechanical losses. Prostheses will equalize leg lengths. Prosthetic fabrication and alignment can be used to correct or at least improve the malrotation. By alignment and fabrication techniques it is possible to increase the stability of the proximal joints by building in alignment stability. The inadequacy of the proximal musculature is only minimally affected by prosthetic applications.

If one accepts the concept of prosthetic correction of biomechanical losses in this group of congenital skeletal limb deficiencies, then treatment must be related to the nature of the defect and to the type of prosthetic restoration that is desired.

UNILATERAL CASES

If one first considers the unilateral cases, the possibilities of treatment are with either a below-knee- or an above-knee-type prosthesis. Except for possible hip surgery, treatment considerations and procedures are essentially the same for all unilateral types.

A unilateral case treated as a below-knee amputee will generally require the Van Nes (*13*) 180-deg tibial rotational osteotomy. By such a procedure the ankle joint becomes the knee joint, and the rotated foot becomes the below-knee stump. This is a procedure which is recommended by many authorities. This author has had no personal experience with it. In selected cases there may be enough femoral length to fit the limb with a below-knee prosthesis without rotation osteotomy, using the anatomical knee joint. In this entity such cases are rare, however.

If one elects to treat a unilateral case as an above-knee-amputee type, then there are several mechanisms by which this type of management may be accomplished.

Without surgical conversion, an above-knee type of prosthesis may be fitted around the deformed foot. The knee joint is mounted below the foot, and by prosthetic fabrication and alignment the axis of rotation is related properly to the line of progression of the patient. Such a procedure generally produces an above-knee socket with a rather bulky distal end, but this bulk can be accommodated by clothing alterations, and the fitting does provide very satisfactory functional restoration.

An alternative procedure is to ablate the foot by ankle disarticulation and fashion a Syme's-type stump closure. This procedure produces an above-knee type of stump of a more satisfactory shape and one which will permit at least partial if not complete end-bearing. A standard knee joint is then attached to the above-knee socket, and by alignment techniques the knee joint is properly related to the line of progression of the patient. This fitting also produces a very satisfactory functional result.

In association with ankle disarticulation, additional surgical conversion procedures may be introduced. Specifically, arthrodesis of the knee will produce a more stable stump skeleton, and in selected cases is a desirable procedure.

In the 30 cases of unilateral PFFD treated at the Area Child Amputee Center, surgical procedures used were as follows: 15 ankle disarticulations, 6 knee arthrodeses, and 7 reconstructions about the hip.

UNILATERAL CASE PRESENTATIONS

The patient depicted in Figure 9-A presents the characteristic clinical appearance of a unilateral PFFD. Prior to admission to the Area Child Amputee Program the patient had been fitted with a shoe and skate that simply equalized leg lengths (Figure 9-B). The patient and his family were not entirely satisfied with his fitting. It was recommended that he be treated by ankle disarticulation and fitting as an above-knee amputee, but he elected to be fitted around the foot. In Figure 9-C the boy is shown wearing a nonstandard prosthesis of a type which can be fitted around the foot of a surgically untreated PFFD. The knee joint is mounted underneath the heel. A standard shinpiece and a SACH foot are used. Figure 9-D presents a close-up view of the hinged split socket of laminated plastic held in place by Velcro straps.

Figure 10-A shows another child with unilateral PFFD. Initial prosthetic fitting was simply to equalize leg lengths by means of an ischial-bearing brace (Figure 10-B). Later, ankle disarticulation with construction of a Syme's-type flap was accomplished (Figure 10-C). The patient was subsequently fitted with a nonstandard above-knee type of prosthesis (Figure 10-D). Early suspension was accomplished by an over-the-shoulder strap; later, simply by a Silesian bandage. Standard knee joints, a standard shankpiece, and a SACH foot are incorporated in the prosthesis.

Figure 11 shows a patient treated by ankle disarticulation and then, in order to give him a more stable above-knee stump, knee arthrodesis.

When knee-joint arthrodesis is to be performed, the time to do this surgery must be carefully selected so that the growth potentials of the proximal tibial and distal femoral epiphyses are not destroyed at too early a date. Miscalculation may produce an above-knee type of stump which is too short for satisfactory prosthetic fitting. Knee-joint arthrodesis helps to correct the flexion, abduction, and external rotation deformities of the hip. These patients can be fitted with standard quadrilateral suction sockets, and end-bearing can sometimes be used if the Syme's-type flap covering the ankle disarticulation has been properly constructed.

In properly selected cases, reconstructive surgical procedures about the hip joint to improve hip stability and thus facilitate maximum usage of hip musculature are desirable. As previously emphasized, only Class A and Class B PFFD cases have adequate acetabula and femoral heads. Hence, it is only in these two groups that reconstructive surgery about the hip would seem to be indicated. It is, therefore, essential that the four radiologic subclasses of the basic clinical entity be clearly differentiated and that hip surgery be carried out only in those cases where there is a femoral head and an acetabulum.

Although the author has himself had experience with the procedure, the best example of reconstructive hip surgery he has seen was a case of the late Dr. Oskar Hepp of Muenster, Germany (11). Figure 12-A shows the preoperative x-ray revealing a typical Class A PFFD. Dr. Hepp simply explored the area and with sharp dissection removed all of the cartilaginous model that existed between the shaft and the head. He then placed the shaft directly underneath the head and held it in 180 deg of valgus until healing occurred. Figure 12-B shows the result three years after surgery.

BILATERAL CASES

It is the author's contention that a patient with bilateral PFFD should not be fitted as a below-knee amputee because bilateral Van Nes rotational osteotomies are not indicated. A patient with bilateral PFFD can walk comfortably and adequately on his own feet. His condition makes him a disproportionate dwarf, but in the confines of his own home he is very apt to ambulate in this manner because he is more stable and comfortable. If one attempts to treat him as a below-knee type by surgical conversion, his ability to ambulate without prostheses is destroyed. If one attempts to fit him as an above-knee amputee and ablate the feet, carry out knee arthrodeses, and do reconstructive surgery about the hip, he is again prevented from ambulating without prostheses. It is the author's firm belief that, in the bilateral case, one should never destroy the patient's ability to ambulate without prostheses. If one accepts this concept, then the prosthetic treatment of children with bilateral PFFD is to fit around the feet, mount the knee joints under the feet, and treat the patient as a bilateral, nonstandard above-knee amputee. Knee arthrodesis is not indicated in these cases because it interferes with nonprosthetic ambulation.

It should be emphasized that the bilateral PFFD's observed in the Area Child Amputee Center have been, with one exception, all Class D cases. Hence, these patients had no acetabula and no femoral heads. Reconstruction about the hip in these cases is probably not indicated. Moreover, if one accepts the concept that these patients desire to walk on their own feet (at least within the confines of their own homes), then arthrodesis of the knees in the presence of severely unstable hips will not improve function.

PRESENTATION OF BILATERAL CASES

The patient shown in Figure 13-A has bilateral PFFD. Since these patients are capable of walking on their own extremities at all times, prosthetic application simply makes it possible for them to be as tall as their contemporaries if they are willing to become "stilt-walkers." Figure 13-B shows this patient with her prostheses. She accommodated to stilt-walking and preferred this method of ambulation out of the confines of her own home. She is shown as a mid-teenager in Figure 13-C. She still walks as an above-knee amputee with her prostheses fitted around her feet. However, she reverts to walking without her prostheses in the confines of her own home, where the disproportionate dwarfism is not the cosmetic problem that it is in public.

Figure 14-A presents a patient with bilateral PFFD who was first seen in infancy in the late 1930's. At that time, the concept of prosthetic application to improve function and cosmesis in bilateral PFFD patients was not recognized. When this patient was approximately fifteen years old, she was recalled and an attempt was made to fit her with stilt-type prostheses, which she rejected. She had adjusted to her disproportionate dwarfism and preferred the stability of walking on her own legs and feet to the instability of walking on the stilt-type prostheses. Figure 14-B shows this patient, now an adult, with her normal son standing beside her. Had this patient been treated by bilateral ankle disarticulation she would have been compelled permanently to walking with prostheses. Given the choice of being a disproportionate dwarf or a stilt-walker, or combining these states, she has had a more satisfactory functional existence. In this instance, she was functional to the point that she has been able to rear a child.

Another bilateral PFFD, shown in Figure 15-A, has associated upper-extremity amelia. He ambulates independently on his own feet. Most patients with bilateral above-knee-type prostheses require some form of external support. The author's figures indicate that 51.7 percent have other limb deficiencies in addition to PFFD. Had this patient been treated by ankle disarticulations he would have been a poor bilateral above-knee prosthetic walker because he has only one upper extremity to utilize for crutch or cane support. This boy was fitted around his feet as an above-knee amputee (Figure 15-B). This gives him normal height if he desires it, but it lets him be independent on his own feet when he desires to be that way.

The patient shown in Figure 16-A had multiple operative procedures in attempts to correct his deformities, and some of these procedures were done about the hip joint. The purpose of these operative procedures was to stabilize the hip joint by iliofemoral arthrodesis in order to increase stability at the hips. An x-ray of the patient's pelvis (Figure 16-B) reveals multiple internal fixation devices. He has ended up with his hips fixed by scar or bony arthrodesis in flexion, abduction, and external rotation, and this fixed position makes it impossible for him to walk without a walker type of external support. He has associated upper-limb anomalies. It is the author's contention that such surgery has not improved this boy's function.

SUMMARY

Proximal femoral focal deficiency is a congenital skeletal limb deficiency involving the proximal end of the femur and, in most instances, the iliofemoral joint. The life history of this anomaly is fairly well known and documented. Serial study of radiographs of these cases indicates that there are four radiographic types. The biomechanical loss in these cases can be categorized as inequality of leg lengths, malrotation, instability of proximal joints, and inadequacy of proximal musculature. Prosthetic application can correct the major biomechanical losses by equalizing leg lengths, correcting malrotation by prosthetic fabrication and alignment, improving the stability of the proximal joint by alignment and fabrication techniques, and at least ameliorating the inadequacy of proximal musculature by prosthetic stability. Classes A and B may obtain improved function by surgical reconstruction about the hip joint. Patients with unilateral PFFD may be treated as below-knee or above-knee amputation-type patients. If they are treated as below-knee patients, they will require a Van Nes 180-deg tibial rotational osteotomy. If they are fitted as above-knee amputees, above-knee prostheses may be fitted around their deformed feet with a knee joint mounted below the foot, a standard shankpiece, and a SACH foot. The alternative is ablation of the foot by ankle disarticulation and the fashioning of a Syme's-type closure. Supplemental knee arthrodesis may be of value. In the bilateral cases, it is the author's contention that patients should be fitted around the deformity so that their feet and knees are preserved in order that they may retain their ability to stand and walk without their prostheses if they so desire, and may have the option of utilizing prostheses for cosmetic restoration as much or as little as they desire.

ACKNOWLEDGMENT

The courtesy of Chester A. Swinyard, M.D., in releasing for publication some of the illustrative material in this monograph is appreciated.

REFERENCES

1. Aitken, G. T. Amputation as a treatment for certain lower extremity congenital abnormalities. J. Bone Joint Surg., 41A (7):1267–1285, 1959.
2. Aitken, G. T. Proximal femoral focal deficiency. *In* Limb Development and Deformity: Problems of Evaluation and Rehabilitation. Springfield, Illinois: Charles C Thomas, Publishers, 1969.
3. Amstutz, H. C., and P. D. Wilson, Jr. Dysgenesis of the proximal femur (coxa vara) and its surgical management. J. Bone Joint Surg. 44A(1):1–24, 1962.
4. Babb, F. S., R. K. Ghormley, and C. C. Chatterton. Congenital coxa vara. J. Bone Joint Surg. 31A(1):115–131, 1949.
5. Fairbank, H. A. T. Infantile or cervical coxa vara, pp. 225–241. *In* The Robert Jones Birthday Volume. London: Oxford University Press, 1928.
6. Frantz, C. H., and R. O'Rahilly. Congenital skeletal limb deficiencies. J. Bone Joint Surg. 43A(8):1202–1224, 1961.
7. Golding, F. C. Congenital coxa vara. J. Bone Joint Surg. 30B(1):161–163, 1948.
8. Golding. F. C. Congenital coxa vara and the short femur. Proc. Roy. Soc. Med. 32:641–648, 1939.
9. Gould, G. M., and W. L. Pyle. Anomalies and Curiosities of Medicine. New York: The Julian Press, Inc., 1896.
10. Hall, C. B., M. B. Brooks, and J. F. Dennis. Congenital skeletal deficiencies of the extremities: Classification and fundamentals of treatment. J.A.M.A. 181:590–599, 1962.
11. Hepp, O. Personal communication.
12. Mital, M. A., K. S. Masalawalla, and M. G. Desai. Bilateral congenital aplasia of the femur. J. Bone Joint Surg. 45B (3):561–565, 1963.
13. Van Nes, C. P. Rotation-plasty for congenital defects of the femur. J. Bone Joint Surg. 32B:12, 1950.

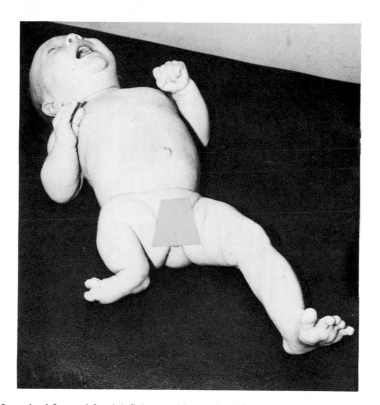

FIGURE 1   Clinical picture of proximal femoral focal deficiency with associated fibular hemimelia. The short femoral segment is flexed, abducted, and externally rotated. The equino-valgus deformity of the foot is typical of fibular hemimelia.

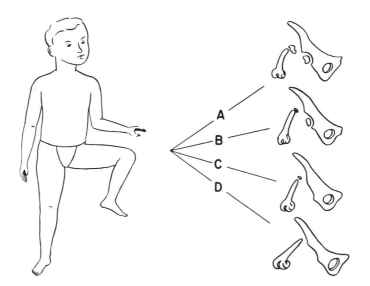

FIGURE 2   Schematic representation of the four radiographic subclasses of proximal femoral focal deficiency.

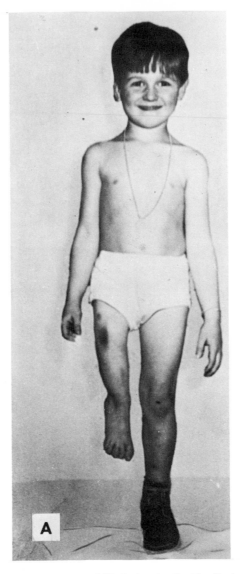

FIGURE 3-A   Clinical picture of PFFD, Class A, with associated fibular hemimelia. The flexion, abduction, and external rotation of the femur are not as severe as usual.

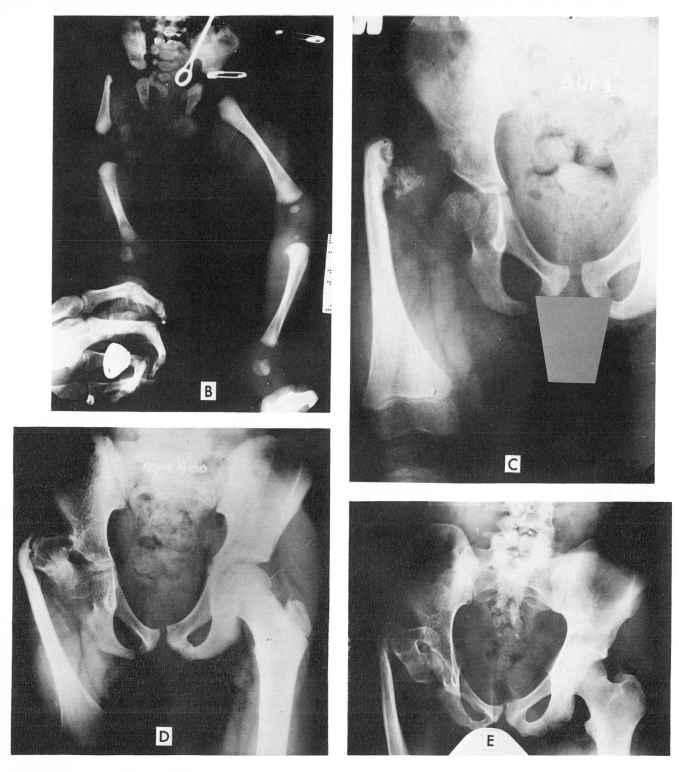

FIGURE 3-B   X-ray of Class A PFFD, age one day. Note short femur with marked lateral displacement proximally and associated fibular hemimelia.

FIGURE 3-C   At six years of age, the x-ray shows an adequate acetabulum, an ossified head of the femur, spotty calcification of the cartilaginous neck and trochanters with severe subtrochanteric varus.

FIGURE 3-D   X-ray at twelve years and four months shows ossification of all elements of the proximal femur with severe subtrochanteric varus and persistent pseudarthrosis.

FIGURE 3-E   X-ray at twenty years. Persistent pseudarthrosis at the subtrochanteric area. Ossification of all elements and severe persistent varus.

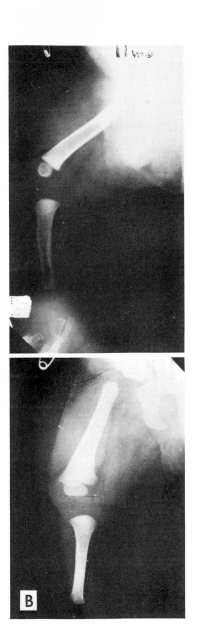

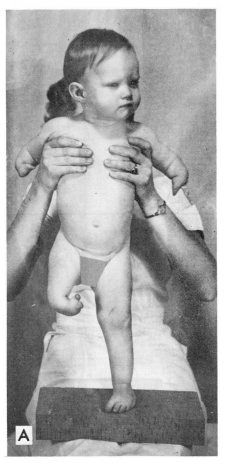

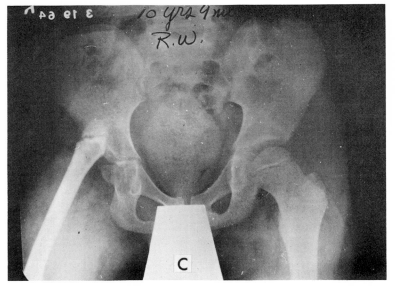

FIGURE 4-A   Clinical manifestations of Class B PFFD.

FIGURE 4-B   X-rays at eleven months show a short femur without ossified head and associated fibular hemimelia.

FIGURE 4-C   An x-ray at ten years and nine months demonstrates the high-riding short femur with ossified head and no evidence of any ossification between head of the femur and proximal end of femoral shaft.

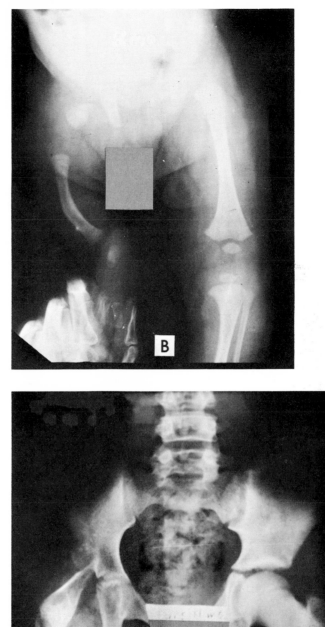

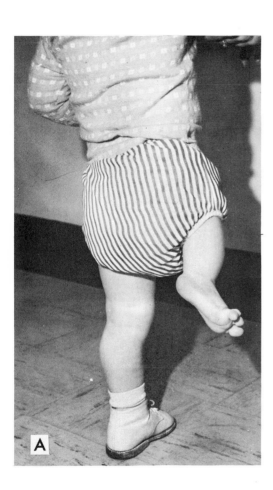

FIGURE 5-A   Clinical picture of Class C PFFD.

FIGURE 5-B   X-ray at two months of age. A short femoral segment is present, but there is no head of the femur. The associated fibular hemimelia is evident.

FIGURE 5-C   X-ray at eleven years and eleven months reveals a severely dysplastic acetabulum, no head of the femur, a high-riding postero-laterally displaced short femoral segment.

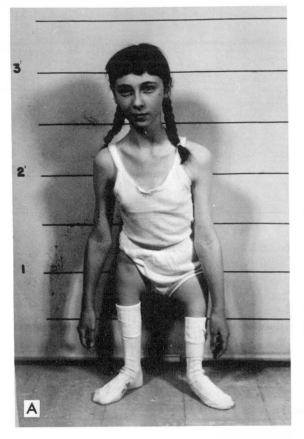

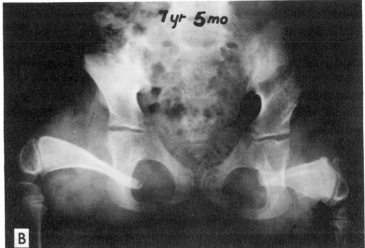

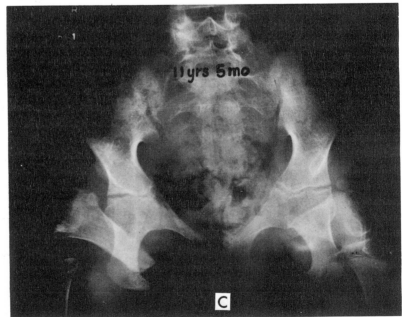

FIGURE 6-A   Clinical picture of bilateral PFFD, Class D.

FIGURE 6-B   X-ray at seven years and five months demonstrates no acetabula, no femoral heads, short, flexed, abducted, externally rotated femoral segments, no proximal femoral tufting.

FIGURE 6-C   X-ray at eleven years and five months. Still no acetabula, no heads of the femurs, and persistent severe flexion, abduction, and external rotation of the femoral segments.

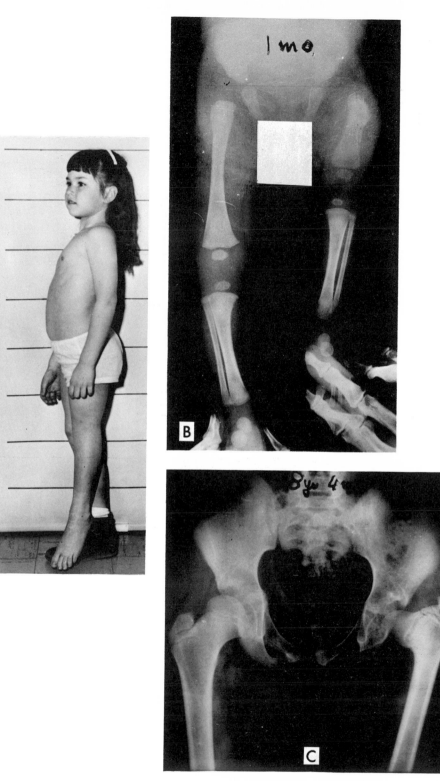

FIGURE 7-A   Clinical picture of inequality of leg lengths with major discrepancy in the femoral segment.

FIGURE 7-B   X-ray at one month of age demonstrates abnormally short femur with lateral displacement and no ossification of the femoral head.

FIGURE 7-C   X-ray at eight years and four months demonstrates changes characteristic of infantile coxa vara.

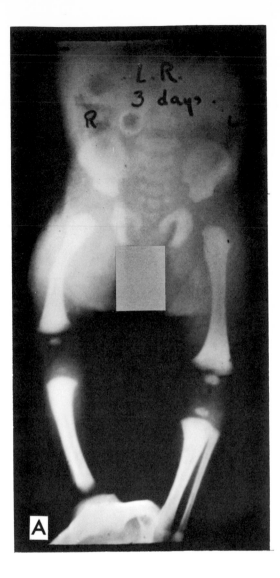

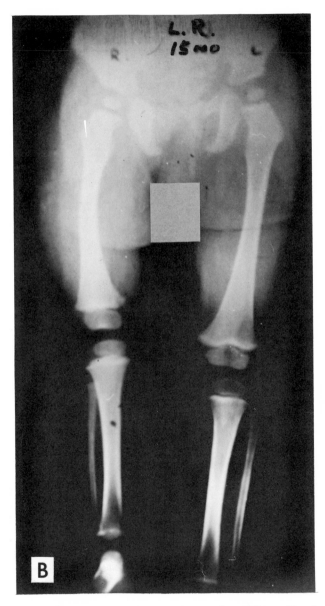

FIGURE 8-A   X-rays of a three-day-old infant demonstrate short femoral and tibial segments; midshaft anterolateral femoral bowing.
FIGURE 8-B   X-ray at fifteen months reveals an essentially normal femur except that it is short. Some minimal shortening of the tibia. Previously noted anterolateral bow has spontaneously undergone nearly complete correction.

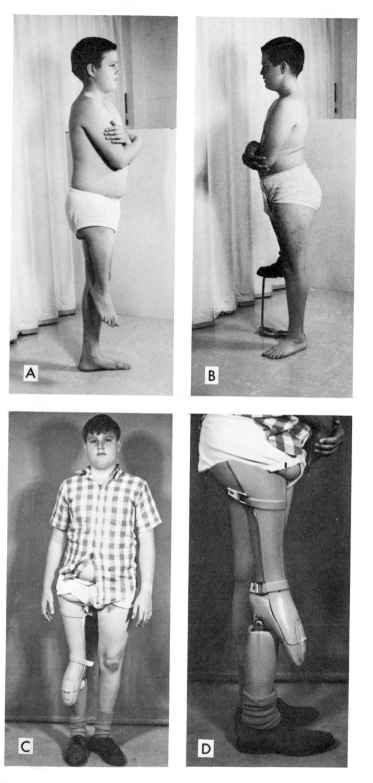

FIGURE 9-A   Clinical picture of unilateral PFFD at twelve years of age.
FIGURE 9-B   Patient was treated initially by shoe and skate shoe lift.
FIGURE 9-C   Patient was fitted with a nonstandard above-knee prosthesis fitted around his deformity.
FIGURE 9-D   Close-up of the hinged anterior panel of the nonstandard above-knee prosthesis, secured with Velcro straps. Note mounting of the knee joint under his heel, with standard shankpiece and SACH foot.

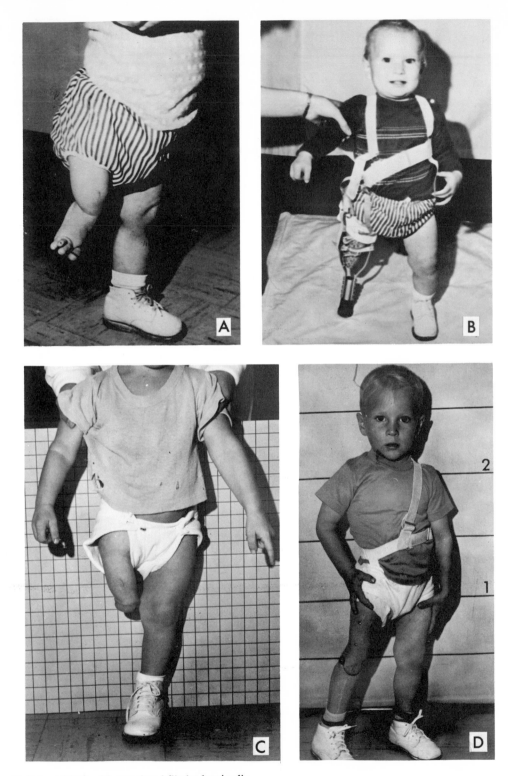

FIGURE 10-A   Unilateral PFFD with associated fibular hemimelia.
FIGURE 10-B   Initial fitting with ischial-bearing pylon with belt and over-the-shoulder strap suspension. Leg lengths have been equalized
 and bipedal ambulation made possible.
FIGURE 10-C   Same patient following ankle disarticulation and construction of a Syme's-type heel flap.
FIGURE 10-D   Same patient fitted with nonstandard above-knee prosthesis with belt and initial over-the-shoulder strap suspension.

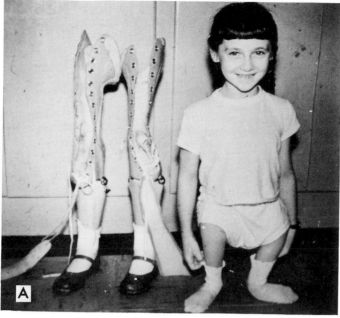

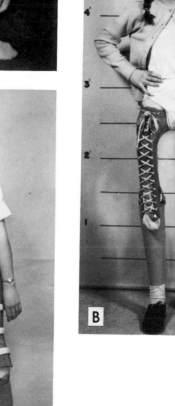

FIGURE 13-A   Bilateral Class D PFFD. This patient has the ability to stand and ambulate comfortably with or without her prostheses.
FIGURE 13-B   Same patient in nonstandard above-knee prostheses fitted around the deformities.
FIGURE 13-C   This patient, seventeen years of age, is now fitted with bilateral nonstandard above-knee prostheses. The prostheses are laminated plastic with an anterior panel secured by Velcro, an improvement over the previous molded leather front-lacer thigh sections.

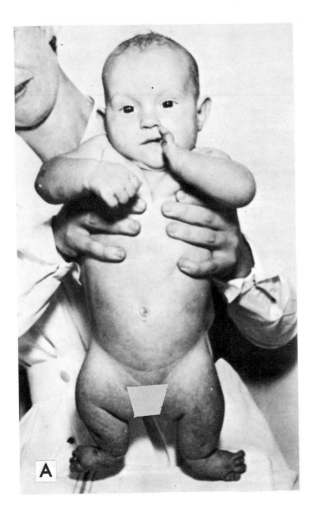

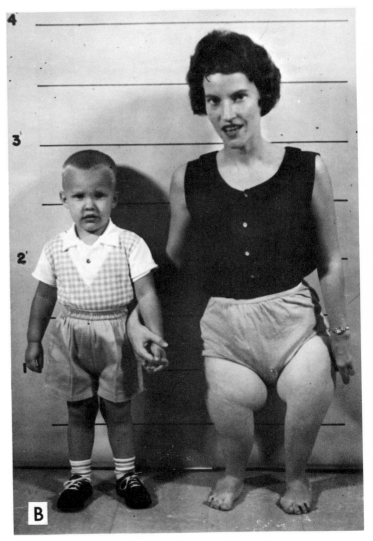

FIGURE 14-A   Bilateral Class D PFFD.
FIGURE 14-B   Same patient at twenty-seven years of age, with her normal son. This patient retains comfortable, secure ambulation without
prostheses.

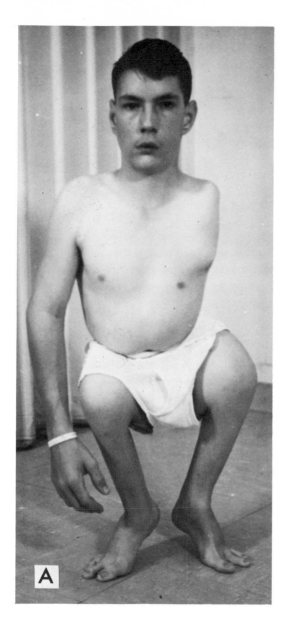

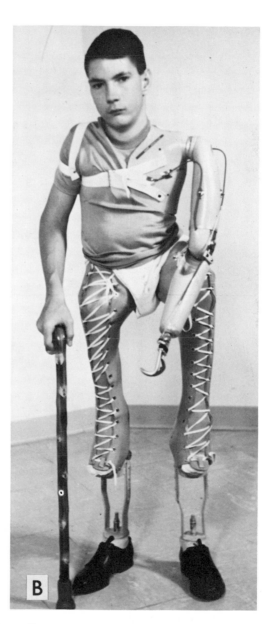

FIGURE 15-A   Bilateral PFFD, Type D, with unilateral upper-extremity amelia.
FIGURE 15-B   Same patient fitted with nonstandard above-knee prostheses and shoulder-disarticulation prosthesis on the amelic upper
    extremity.

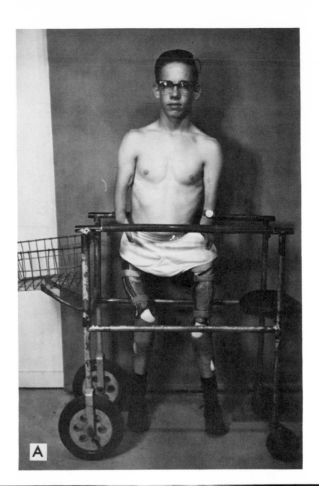

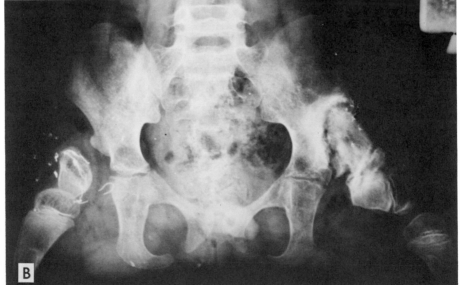

FIGURE 16-A   Bilateral PFFD, Type D, with associated upper-extremity anomalies. He was fitted with nonstandard above-knee prostheses and ambulated with the assistance of a walker.

FIGURE 16-B   An x-ray of the patient reveals evidences of multiple surgical procedures directed toward producing iliofemoral arthrodeses and permitting knee joints to substitute for hip joints. Final position of the femoral segments has not corrected undesirable flexion, abduction, and external rotation of the femurs.

RICHARD E. KING, M.D.

Some Concepts of
PROXIMAL FEMORAL FOCAL DEFICIENCY

*Whenever a large sample of chaotic elements is taken in hand
and marshalled in order of their magnitude, an unsuspected
and most beautiful form of regularity proves to have been
latent all along.*

—GALTON, *Natural Inheritance,* 1889

By definition, the term "proximal femoral focal deficiency"
implies that the proximal femur is lacking in completeness.
That this incompleteness is only part of the problem was
made clear by the study of many x-rays in an attempt to
cull true cases of this type from the morass of what has been
frequently classified as proximal femoral focal deficiency.
A study of the past literature has also revealed that not un-
commonly cases of congenital short femur, epiphyseal coxa
vara, and phocomelia have been included with the PFFD
group (*3, 18, 20, 25, 31, 45, 48, 51, 52, 59*).

CLASSIFICATION OF TYPES

It remained for Aitken (*1*) to present a workable classification that is easily understood and that can serve as a background for the surgical correction of this condition (Figure 1).
As seen in Figure 2, Types A and B show elements of the
proximal femur, i.e., acetabulum and head; whereas Types
C and D show no evidence of acetabulum and consequently
no head or neck of the femur. These four types all present
clinically with a thigh that has the appearance of a ship's
funnel and is almost always flexed, abducted, and externally
rotated (Figure 3). It is not uncommon for the ankle on the
affected side to lie at the level of the knee joint on the normal
side. Complete absence of the fibula on the affected side is
frequently associated with proximal femoral focal deficiencies. Nilsonne (*45*) reports a 50 percent incidence,
Aitken (*1*) 70 percent, and Amstutz (*2*) 80 percent.

EMBRYOLOGY

Ossification is commonly delayed in congenital deformities,
and this delay is seen in proximal femoral focal deficiency
also.

Because of the delayed ossification of the femoral head,
ingenious attempts to attain pelvi-femoral stability by bone
graft from the shaft of the femur to the acetabulum have
been described in the literature (*35, 50, 52*). Lloyd-Roberts
(*38*) performed arthrography in two cases in order to outline
the process of delayed femoral head ossification, which was
present in both of his cases.

Much of this confusion can be resolved when we realize
that the ilium and proximal femur develop from a common
cartilage anlage. The elements of head and neck of the femur
are actually hewn from this common block of cartilage, and
the hip joint appears as a cleft between the head of the femur
and what is later the acetabulum (*19, 30, 32, 36, 47, 56, 57*).

Laurenson (*36*) states that the head of the femur and the
acetabulum gradually separate from each other by formation
of a cleft and then formation of a definitive joint cavity. At
nine weeks the embryonic hip joint resembles the general
form of the adult.

Figure 4-A represents a 17-mm embryo and shows the
approximate size of the limb bud. The development of the
hip joint at this stage is shown in Figures 4-B and 4-C. The
ilium, ischium, and pubis still consist of precartilage, and
the acetabulum shows little increase in its concavity. By

this time the head of the femur is slightly rounded, and while the acetabulum is not much more concave than in younger specimens, there is nevertheless a slight depression more marked medially which contains loose tissue and indicates a primitive acetabular fossa (19, 56, 57).

At 22 mm (Figures 5-A, 5-B, and 5-C), the acetabulum deepens medially. Both trochanters are now well defined, but the neck of the femur is short. Note the beginning of cavitation at the periphery of the interzone where dissolution is occurring to form the acetabular cleft. As chondrification proceeds in the blastemal anlage, the portion of the blastema between femur and acetabulum remains unchondrified to form a disc or interzone. However, at 20 mm its middle portion becomes lighter in staining density and a three-layered arrangement is evident (19, 56, 57).

At 30 mm (Figures 6-A through 6-D), the acetabular cavity is well developed, but obliterated at the center. Figures 7-A through 7-E trace embryological development in fetuses from 73 to 270 mm. Figure 7-A shows the acetabular fossa, fovea capitis femoris, and early vascularization at the femoral neck and near the glenoid lip at 73 mm. In Figure 7-B, at 106 mm, vascularization is considerably advanced and ligaments are well defined. Figure 7-C shows increased ossification and vascularization at 180 mm. Figure 7-D, at 250 mm, depicts the proximal extent of diaphyseal ossification. At 270 mm, the fovea capitis, filled with vascular tissue sharply demarcated from cartilage, is shown in Figure 7-E (19, 56, 57).

A composite of fetuses from 44 mm to 126 mm is shown in Figure 8 to indicate the relative external appearance of the lower extremity.

Since the lower limb develops in a proximodistal direction, and in view of the embryological development described above, may we not infer that if an acetabulum is visualized at birth a femoral head will appear? Conversely, may we not assume that if no acetabulum is present at birth no elements of proximal femur will appear?

This conclusion has been corroborated in our review of x-rays on over 100 cases of proximal femoral focal deficiency collected from various juvenile amputee clinics throughout the United States. When we establish that a femoral head is present, although delayed in ossification, our attempts at surgical correction can be initiated earlier and without confusion as to whether or not a femoral head is present (33, 34).

We can only postulate that the cause of this error of development is some type of insult sustained by the embryonic lower extremity at the time that the cleft which later represents the hip joint is being formed. Whether this insult is some transient physical or chemical trauma to the limb bud at this stage, we are not prepared to say (61, 62). It is significant that Duraiswami (15), injecting insulin into the yolk sac on the sixth day of the developing chick embryo, was able to produce some deficiency of the proximal femur (Figures 9-A and 9-B).

TREATMENT

CONSERVATIVE

The nonstandard prosthesis typically fitted to all types of patients with uncorrected proximal femoral focal deficiency usually includes a wide-mouthed socket, a platform for support of the foot, and outside knee joints (Figures 10-A and 10-B). Functionally and cosmetically this prosthesis leaves much to be desired.

SURGICAL

General Principles

Because of dissatisfaction with the results of conservative management, an attempt has been made to convert surgically the existing elements of the femur to a single skeletal lever so that a standard conventional prosthesis could be used.

The usual deformity presented is one of external rotation, flexion, and abduction of the proximal portion of the femur. The surgery performed usually does not require that special attention be directed to these contractures, i.e., surgery directed toward completion and achievement of an intact skeletal lever usually is sufficient to correct the contracture about the hip area.

Analysis of the skin, nerves, bone, joint, and musculature of a proximal femoral focal deficiency reveals that a single skeletal lever with adequate skin, no disturbance of the nerves or circulation, adequate bone, good joint function, and musculature sufficient to move the skeletal lever can be achieved surgically. In providing a skeletal lever, every effort should be made to provide pelvi-femoral stability also.

It cannot be emphasized too frequently or strongly that each individual case requires careful analysis if an appropriate solution to this formidable problem is to be found. Also, the surgeon must be aware that if an acetabulum is present at birth, elements of a femoral head will eventually develop. Awareness of this developmental sequence will obviate unnecessary attempts at obtaining pelvi-femoral stability by such means as bifurcation, osteotomies, and bone grafts (34, 50, 52).

Specific Surgical Techniques for Each of the Four Types of Proximal Femoral Focal Deficiency in the Aitken Classification

Type A   Type A proximal femoral focal deficiency can be realigned by osteotomy for better mechanical leverage. This procedure should be done at the subtrochanteric level, and the osteotomy site can be held by internal fixation, pins, etc. A case in point is that of B.B., who was first seen at the age of nine months. X-rays revealed a Type A proximal femoral focal deficiency (Figure 11-A). At eighteen months x-rays revealed developing varus with bending occurring at the subtrochanteric level (Figure 11-B). An osteotomy was done at the subtrochanteric level and fixed at 90 deg in a spica cast. Subsequent healing is shown in Figure 11-C. When the patient was last seen, in May 1968, x-rays revealed complete remodeling of the proximal femur (Figure 11-D). Clinical photographs of the stump and of the patient in his prosthesis were made at this time (Figures 11-E and 11-F).

Type B   Type B proximal femoral focal deficiency requires realignment of the fragments to create a skeletal lever. Two case reports demonstrate a planned approach to the achievement of this end.

P.M., initially seen at the age of 2½ years, presented the flexion, external rotation, and abduction of hip deformities typical of proximal femoral focal deficiency (Figures 12-A and 12-B). This patient had never walked because of lack of stability in the hip area. An attempt was made to align the skeletal fragments over an intramedullary rod.

The area of pseudarthrosis between the neck of the femur and the elements of the distal femur and its epiphysis was removed (Figure 13). This was good cartilage in a dormant state of endochondral ossification, and mere realignment of the fragments in a semblance of weight-bearing position was sufficient to awaken it so that normal endochondral ossification could ensue (Figure 14) (*8, 51, 52, 59*).

Figure 15 shows the fragments of the proximal and distal femur fixed over an intramedullary rod, with the rod presented distally in the region of the foot.

A knee arthrodesis was performed, concomitant with the realignment of the femoral segments (Figure 16).

Figure 17 shows the final realignment of knee fusion and pseudarthrosis to make a single skeletal lever.

Approximately two months later a disarticulation at the ankle was performed. The knee fusion was solid and the intramedullary rod was removed at the time of the disarticulation (Figure 18). This procedure retains intact the epiphyses of the distal femur and proximal and distal tibia. It is noteworthy that the ankle disarticulation at this age provides a stump the distal end of which is level with the opposite knee for a cosmetic prosthetic application (Figures 19-A, 19-B, and 19-C).

With the skeletal lever stabilized, the range of motion and strength available for prosthetic control is quite impressive (Figures 20-A, 20-B, and 20-C). The patient was fitted with a conventional thigh-corset prosthesis with hip control (Figures 21-A and 21-B).

At present, this patient plays on a soccer team and is active in every phase of everyday childhood life. Sufficient time has not yet elapsed for proper evaluation of the epiphyses of the distal femur and proximal and distal tibia. However, the latest x-rays on this boy, taken in January 1967, still show the epiphyses to be open, and 2 cm of growth have occurred in the single skeletal segment (Figure 22).

P.D. was initially seen shortly after her birth on September 29, 1960, and was followed through the Georgia Crippled Children's Service. The child's thigh had the typical ship's-funnel appearance, with the usual flexion, external rotation, and abduction contractures (Figure 23-A). The patient was fitted with an extension brace and ambulation was permitted. The child was referred to the Juvenile Amputee Clinic in February 1965, at which time x-rays revealed a Type B proximal femoral focal deficiency (Figure 23-B).

In April 1965, an attempt was made to place the sharpened spike of the distal femur into a mortise in the femoral head (*25, 35, 52*). At the same time a knee fusion was performed. The sequence of procedures was as follows: a 6-mm intramedullary Küntcher rod was driven retrograde through the tibia and out of the foot. The femur was then threaded onto this rod to complete the knee fusion. The rod was driven proximally into the femur. At this time the sharp spike of the femur was placed into the mortise in the femoral head. However, the upper end of the femur was bowed, and the intramedullary rod came out laterally. Therefore, the entire limb was held in 90-deg abduction, and the rod was driven into the anterior inferior spine of the ilium, thus stabilizing the femoral–tibial segments in this position, as well as offering a supporting strut to the epiphyseal-diaphyseal fusion (femoral head to the femoral shaft). The patient was placed in a double spica cast with the affected extremity in 90-deg abduction.

Sections from the proximal femur showed viable cartilage (Figure 24), and sections from the epiphysis of the femoral head showed a viable but somewhat disorganized epiphyseal line (Figure 25). On July 7, 1965, the spica was removed, and x-rays revealed a thin spicule of bone from femur to femoral head (Figure 26). It was felt that this spicule represented a precarious attachment, and another spica was applied for an additional month. When this cast was removed on August 11, 1965, x-rays were made in adduction and abduction, and it was believed that the femur and femoral head moved as a single unit.

By February 15, 1966, the patient had been putting some weight on the foot, and x-rays revealed that the thin spicule of bone had hypertrophied and was now the thickness of a thumb (Figure 27). The knee also appeared to be solid. The intramedullary rod was removed and at the same time a Syme's amputation was performed (Figure 28).

On March 23, 1966, the patient was found to have a stable hip with no flexion contracture (Figure 29). Satisfactory stump abduction, flexion, and extension were present (Figures 30-A through 30-D). On this date the patient was fitted with a plastic funnel-shaped socket with an ischial seat, metal hip control, single-axis knee, and SACH foot (Figures 31-A, 31-B, and 31-C).

The patient received prosthetics training and is now ambulating well. When seen in July of 1966, x-rays revealed further apparent hypertrophy of the proximal femur with a suggestion of increased growth of the femoral head. The patient had developed an inexplicable line of translucency in the femoral shaft (Figure 32). Perhaps this zone represented an area through which bending may occur to cause a subsequent coxa vara. If necessary, osteotomy to realign this bending could be performed later and should cause this zone to close. However, x-rays taken in March 1967 showed this translucent zone to be closing with use of the prosthesis (Figure 33).

Type C   Patients with Type C proximal femoral focal deficiency can only be offered a knee fusion to achieve a skeletal lever since no pelvi-femoral stability exists or can be provided. Since the femur usually presents as a long segment, the ankle joint lies at a level below the knee joint of the normal leg. An example of this type of case is A.R., who was seen shortly after birth (Figures 34-A and 34-B). Subsequent x-rays show surgical fusion of the knee. A below-knee amputation at the level of the opposite knee was done after the knee fusion was solid (Figures 35-A and 35-B). Follow-up two years after amputation has shown no evidence of overgrowth.

Amputation of the affected leg will be at the below-knee level rather than through the ankle in order to bring the prosthetic knee level with the normal knee joint.

Since the distal tibial epiphysis is removed, this amputation should be done as near growth completion as possible to decrease the chance of overgrowth of tibia and fibula.

Type D   Type D proximal femoral focal deficiency presents a formidable problem, and we can only offer our contemplated plans for surgical conversion. Pelvi-femoral stability can be achieved by a preliminary Chiari transinnominate osteotomy. Then the element of the distal femur can be fixed to the pelvic shelf to allow the knee joint to serve as a hip joint. Later a disarticulation of the ankle can be done so that a conventional prosthesis may be worn. We have not as yet tried this procedure, but we feel that sufficient musculature is present to flex and extend the knee joint so that it could be made to act as an effective hip joint (Figures 36-A and 36-B).

CONCLUSIONS

An attempt has been made to use a classification system for proximal femoral focal deficiency developed by Aitken that allows us to proceed to a planned surgical approach for each of the four types identified. Each case should be evaluated separately, and the type of surgical conversion best suited to the elements of the proximal femur present should be performed. It has not been found necessary to correct the contractures present by a separate procedure. In the conversions described in this paper, the contractures of flexion, abduction, and external rotation are probably released through the soft tissue dissection and femoral

shortening associated with the knee fusion which is done at the same time. The principle of establishing a single skeletal lever by alignment of fragments over an intramedullary rod has so far proven sound. It has provided pelvi-femoral and skeletal stability of the femoral segment upon which existing musculature can act to operate a prosthesis. Although this is a preliminary report based on six cases of surgical conversion, we have not as yet noticed any closure of epiphyseal lines due to the central penetration of epiphyseal plates by an intramedullary rod. These thoughts are presented in the hopes of stimulating others to an awareness that reasonable function, comfort, and cosmesis result from this approach to these formidable deformities.

BIBLIOGRAPHY

1. Aitken, G. T. Instructional Course Lecture, American Academy of Orthopaedic Surgeons, 1967.
2. Amstutz, H. C. Personal communication.
3. Amstutz, H. C., and P. D. Wilson, Jr. Dysgenesis of the proximal femur (coxa vara) and its surgical management. J. Bone Joint Surg. 44A(1):1–24, 1962.
4. Arey, L. B. Developmental Anatomy, 6th ed. Philadelphia: W. B. Saunders Company, 1954.
5. Bagg, H. J. Etiology of certain congenital structural defects. Amer. J. Obstet. Gynec. 8:131–141, 1924.
6. Bagg, H. J. Hereditary abnormalities of the limbs, their origin and transmission; ii. A morphological study with special reference to the etiology of club-feet, syndactylism, hypodactylism, and congenital amputation in the descendants of x-rayed mice. Amer. J. Anat. 43:167–219, 1929.
7. Bardeen, C. R., and W. H. Lewis. Development of the limbs, bodywall and back in man. Amer. J. Anat. 1:1–35, 1901.
8. Blenche, Mittheilung aus der orthopädischen Heilanstalt von Dr. Blenche in Magdeburg. Ueber congenitalen Femurdefect. Z. Ortho. Chir. 9:584–656, 1901.
9. Borggreve, J. Kniegelenksersatz durch das in der Beinlängsachse um 180° gedrehte Fussgelenk. Arch. Orthopäd. Chir. 28:175–178, 1930.
10. Breasted, J. H., ed. Edwin Smith Surgical Papyrus. Chicago: University of Chicago Press, 1930 (Vol. 3, Univ. Chicago Oriental Inst. Publications).
11. Burgess, E. The surgical means of obtaining hip stability with motion in congenital proximal femoral deficiency. ICIB I(3):1–4, December 1961.
12. Campbell's Operative Orthopaedics, Vol. 2, pp. 2040-2042 (3rd Ed.). St. Louis, Mo.: The C. V. Mosby Company, 1956.
13. Cohn, I. Skeletal disturbances and anomalies, A clinical report and review of the literature. Radiology 18:592–626, 1932.
14. Colonna, P. C. Some common congenital deformities and their orthopedic treatment. N.Y. State J. Med. 28:713–714, 1928.
15. Duraiswami, P. K. Experimental causation of congenital skeletal defects and its significance in orthopedic surgery. J. Bone Joint Surg. 34B:646–698, 1952.
16. Duraiswami, P. K. Personal communication.
17. Fraser, F. C., and T. D. Fainstal. Causes of congenital defects: Review. Amer. J. Dis. Child. 82:593–603, 1951.
18. Freund, E. Congenital defects of femur, fibula and tibia. Arch. Surg. 33:349–391, 1936.

19. Gardner, E., and D. J. Gray. Prenatal development of the human hip joint. Amer. J. Anat. 87:163–211, 1950.
20. Golding, F. C. Congenital coxa vara and the short femur. Proc. Roy. Soc. Med. 32:641–648, 1939.
21. Golding, F. C. Congenital coxa vara. J. Bone Joint Surg. 30B: 161–163, 1948.
22. Gordon, G. C. Congenital Deformities. Edinburgh: E. & S. Livingstone, Ltd., 1961.
23. Gruenwald, P. Mechanisms of abnormal development. Arch. Path. 44:398–436, 495–559, 648–664, 1947.
24. Gruenwald, P. Developmental pathology; A new field in medicine. Amer. J. Obstet. Gynec. 58:1–14, 1949.
25. Guilleminet, M., L. Michel, and C. R. Michel. Les absences congénitales du fémur. Rev. Chir. Orthopéd. 46:15–46, 1960.
26. Hall, John E. Rotation of congenitally hypoplastic lower limbs to use the ankle joint as a knee. ICIB VI(2):3–9, 1966.
27. Hamilton, W. J., J. D. Boyd, and H. W. Mossman. Human Embryology. Baltimore: Williams and Wilkins, 1952.
28. Haring, O. M., and F. J. Lewis. The etiology of congenital developmental anomalies. Int. Abstr. Surg., S.G.O. 113:1–18, 1961.
29. Harris, H. A. Congenital abnormalities of the skeleton, Chap. 18. *In* The Chances of Morbid Inheritance. C. P. Blacker, ed. London: H. K. Lewis, 1934.
30. Harrison, T. J. The influence of the femoral head on pelvic growth and acetabular form in the rat. J. Anat. 95:12–24, 1961.
31. King, R. E. Concepts of proximal femoral focal deficiencies. ICIB I(2):1–7, 1961.
32. King, R. E. Proximal femoral focal deficiencies. ICIB III(9):1–5, 1964.
33. King, R. E. Surgical correction of proximal femoral focal deficiency. ICIB IV(10):1–10, 1965.
34. King, R. E. Providing a single skeletal lever in proximal femoral focal deficiency. ICIB VI(2):23–28, 1966.
35. Langston, H. H. Congenital defect of the shaft of the femur. Brit. J. Surg. 27:162–165, 1939.
36. Laurenson, R. D. Bilateral anomalous development of the hip joint. Post mortem study of a human fetus, twenty-six weeks old. J. Bone Joint Surg. 46A(2):283–292, 1964.
37. Lewin, P. Congenital absence or defects of bones of the extremities. Amer. J. Roentgenol. 4:431–448, 1917.
38. Lloyd-Roberts, G. C., and K. H. Stone. Congenital hypoplasia of the upper femur. J. Bone Joint Surg. 45B(3):557–560, 1963.
39. Mall, F. P. On ossification centres in human embryos less than one hundred days old. Amer. J. Anat. 5:433–458, 1906.
40. Manohar, K. Congenital absence of the right femur. Brit. J. Surg. 27:158–161, 1931.
41. Meyer, D. M., and W. Swanker. Anomalies of Infants and Children. New York: McGraw-Hill Book Company, 1958.
42. Miller, H. C. Symposium on congenital anomalies: Scope and incidence of congenital abnormalities. Pediatrics 6:320–324, 1950.
43. Murphy, D. P. Congenital Malformations. Philadelphia: J. B. Lippincott Company, 1947.
44. Murphy, D. P. Symposium on orthopedic surgery; congenital malformations. S. Clin. N. Amer. 33:1623–1631, 1953.
45. Nilsonne, H. Über den Kongenitalen Femur Defekt. Arch. Orthopädische Unfall-Chirurgie. 26:138–169, 1928.
46. Ollerenshaw, R. Congenital defects of the long bones of the lower limb. J. Bone Joint Surg. 7:528–552, 1925.
47. O'Rahilly, R. Morphological patterns in limb deficiencies and duplications. Amer. J. Anat. 89:135–194, 1951.
48. Reiner, M. Ueber den Congenitalen Femurdefect. Z. Ortho. Chir. 9:544–583, 1901.
49. Reisner, G. A. The Hearst Medical Papyrus, University of California Publications, Egyptian Archaeology, Vol. I. Leipzig: J. C. Hinricks, 1905.
50. Ring, P. A. Congenital short femur. J. Bone Joint Surg. 41B:73–79, 1959.
51. Ring, P. A. Congenital abnormalities of the femur. Arch. Dis. Child. 36:410–417, 1961.
52. Sideman, S. Agenesis femur–report of case. J. Int. Surg. 40: 152–165, 1963.
53. Smith, G. E., and F. W. Jones. Archaeological Survey of Nubia, Report for 1907–1908. Vol. I and II. Report of Human Remains. Cairo: National Printing Company, 1910.
54. Smith, G. E., and W. R. Dawson. Egyptian Mummies. London: Allen and Unwin, 1924.
55. Stransky, E., and Abad-Vasquez. On congenital malformations of the femur. Ann. Pediat. 200:31–38, 1963.
56. Strayer, L., Jr. Embryology of the hip joint. Yale J. Biol. 16: 1–26, 1943.
57. Strayer, L., Jr. Congenital deformities of lower extremity. A.A.O.S. Proceedings, Vol. VII, 1950.
58. Streeter, G. L. Focal deficiencies in fetal tissues and their relation to intra-uterine amputation. Contributions to Embryology, Carnegie Inst. of Washington 22(414):1–44, 1930.
59. Teal, F. Personal communication.
60. Van Nes, C. P. Rotation-plasty for congenital defects of femur. J. Bone Joint Surg. 32B:12–16, 1950.
61. Warkany, J. Some factors in the etiology of congenital malformations. Amer. J. Ment. Def. 50:231–241, 1945.
62. Warkany, J. Congenital anomalies. Pediatrics. 7:607–610, 1951.

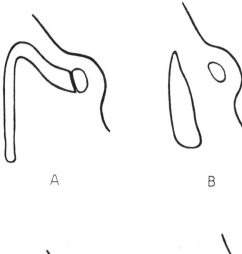

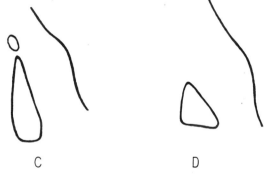

FIGURE 1   Diagrammatic representation of four types of proximal femoral focal deficiency (Aitken).

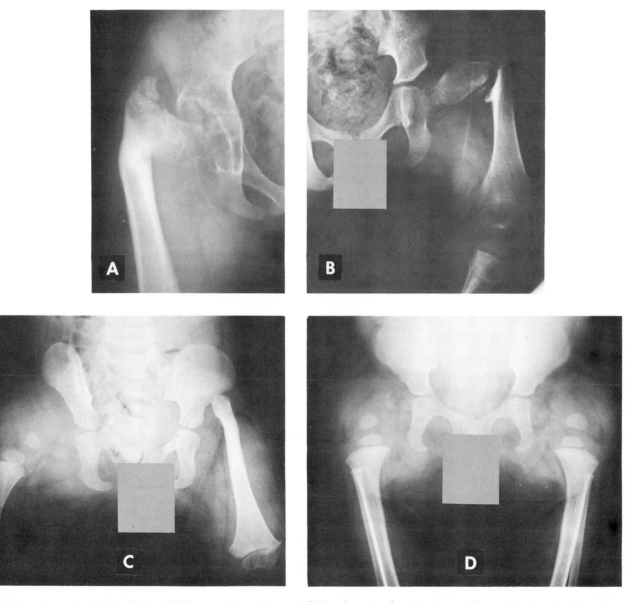

FIGURE 2   Examples of Aitken's four PFFD types. Type A (upper left) has elements of acetabulum and femoral head as does Type B (upper right). Type C (lower left) and Type D (lower right) exhibit lack of acetabulum and head of femur.

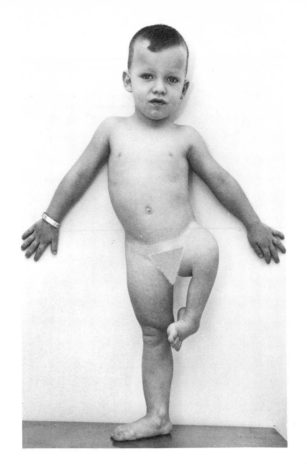

FIGURE 3   Characteristic abduction, flexion, and external rotation of thigh.

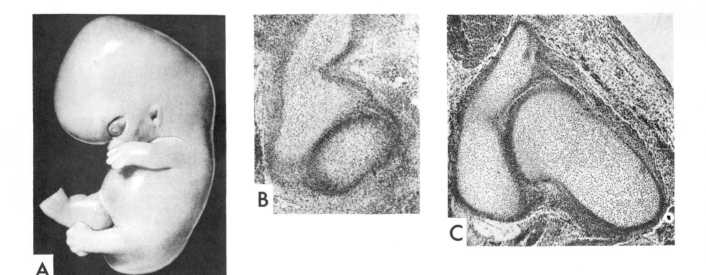

FIGURES 4-A, 4-B, and 4-C   A 17-mm embryo, and development of the hip joint at this stage.

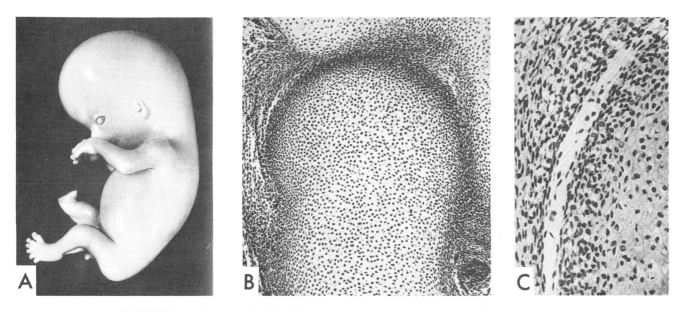

FIGURES 5-A, 5-B, and 5-C   The 22-mm embryo and development of the hip joint at this stage.

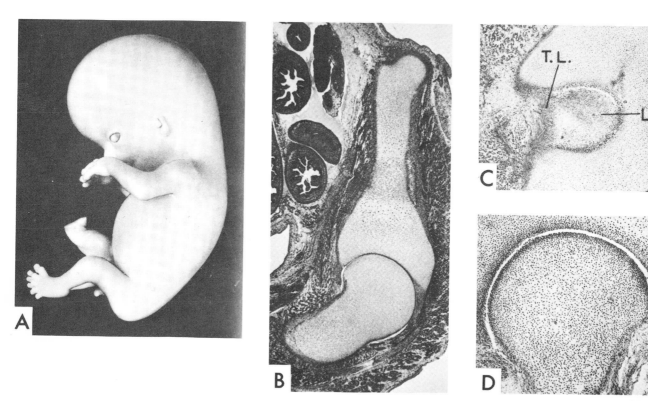

FIGURES 6-A through 6-D   The 30-mm embryo and development of the hip joint at this stage. (L.T., ligament teres; T.L., transverse acetabular ligament.)

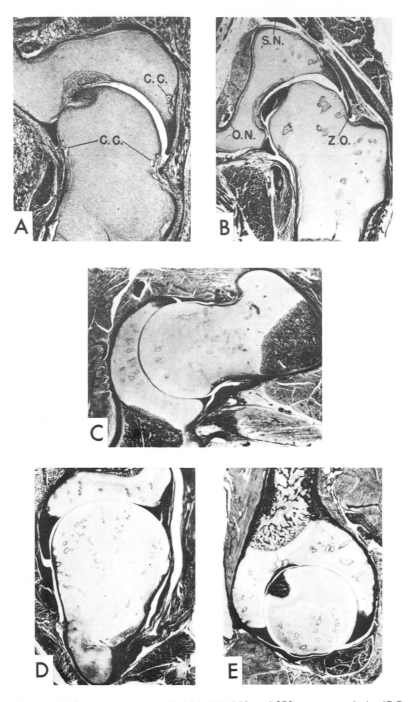

FIGURES 7-A through 7-E   Embryonic hip development at 73, 106, 180, 250, and 270 mm, respectively. (C.C., cartilage canals; O.N., obturator nerve; S.N., sciatic nerve; Z.O., zona orbicularis.

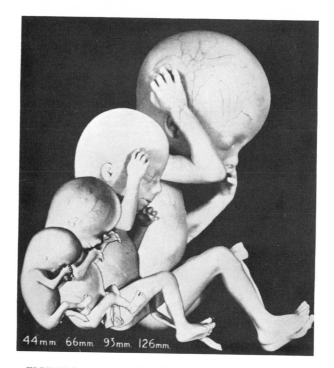

FIGURE 8   A composite of fetuses from 44 to 126 mm.

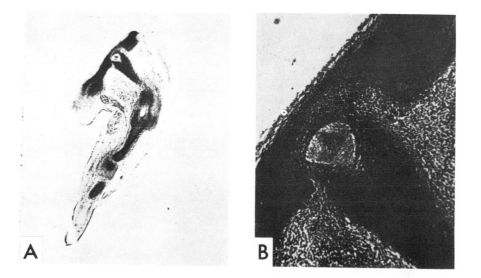

FIGURE 9-A   A sagittal section (×18) of the left hind limb of a seven-day-old insulin-treated chick embryo showing areas of degeneration in the upper ends of the femur and tibia.
FIGURE 9-B   Photomicrograph (×100) to show the degenerative changes in the upper end of the femur.

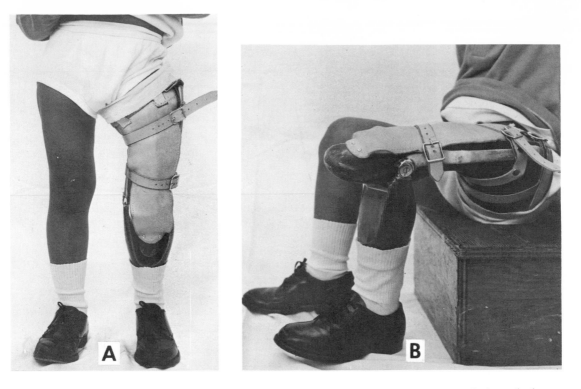

FIGURES 10-A and 10-B   Standing and sitting views of patient with preoperative nonstandard prosthesis.

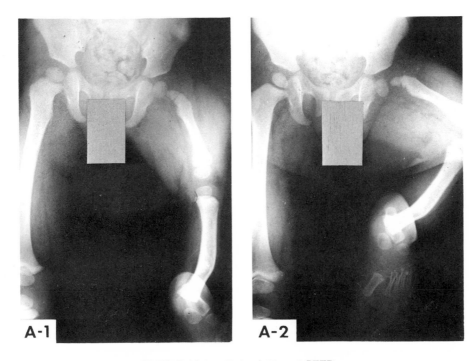

FIGURE 11-A   Patient's Type A PFFD.

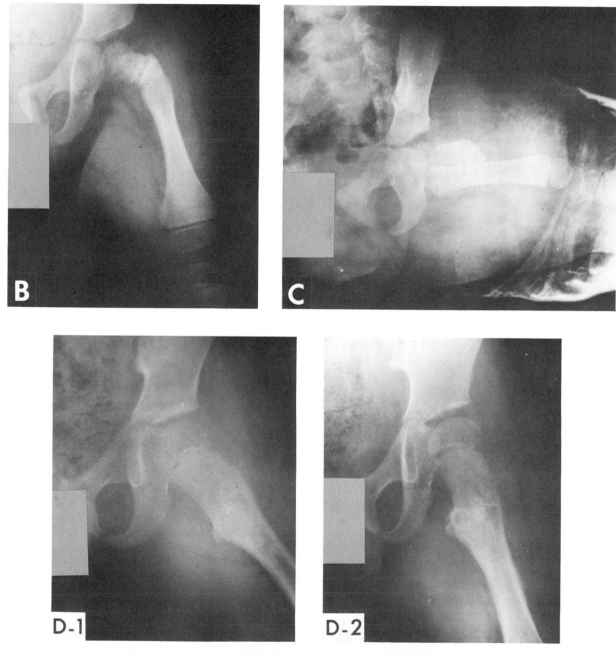

FIGURE 11-B   The development of varus at 18 months.
FIGURE 11-C   Healing following osteotomy at subtrochanteric level.
FIGURE 11-D   May 1968 x-rays showing complete remodeling of proximal femur.

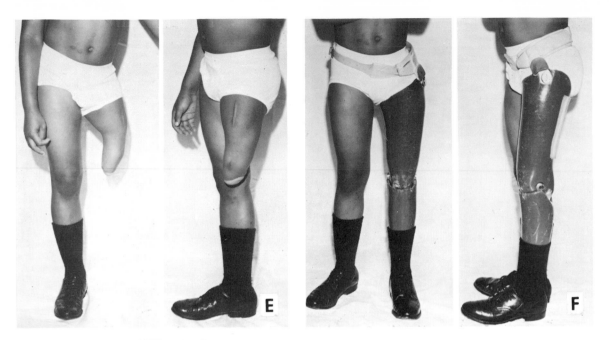

FIGURE 11-E   Anterior and lateral views of stump following removal of foot.
FIGURE 11-F   Anterior and lateral views of postoperative prosthesis.

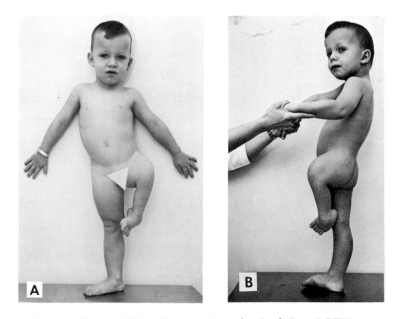

FIGURES 12-A and 12-B   External views of patient's Type B PFFD.

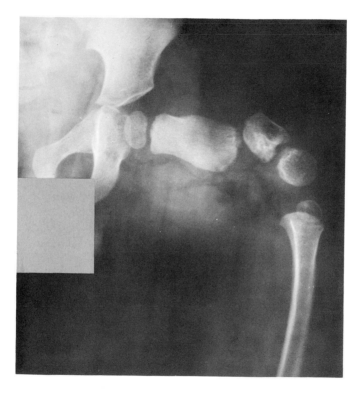

FIGURE 13   Preoperative x-ray of patient's hip joint.

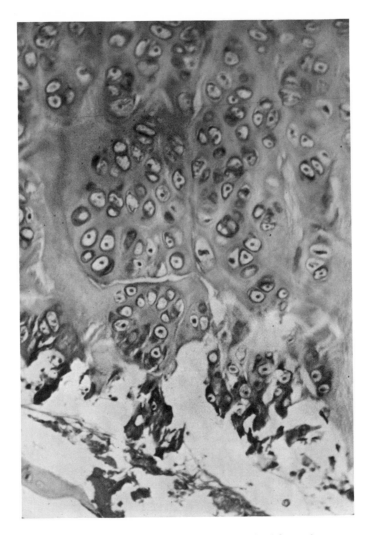

FIGURE 14   Cartilage removed from proximal femoral area.

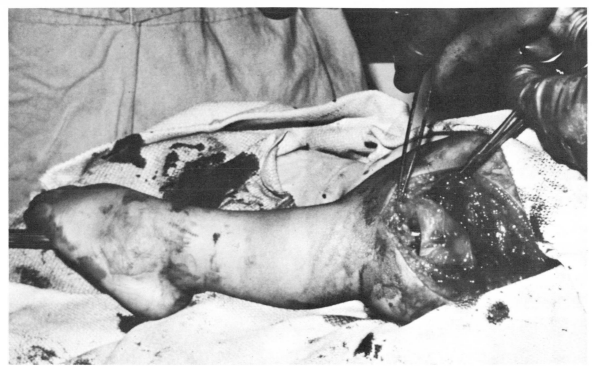

FIGURE 15   Fragments of proximal and distal femur fixed over an intramedullary rod.

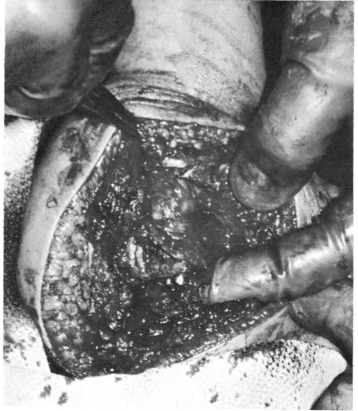

FIGURE 16   Performance of knee arthrodesis.

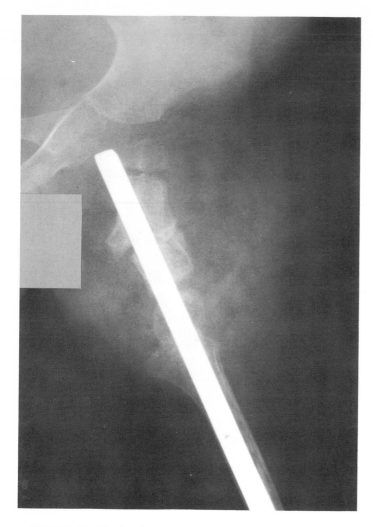

FIGURE 17   Final realignment of knee fusion and pseudarthrosis to make a single skeletal lever.

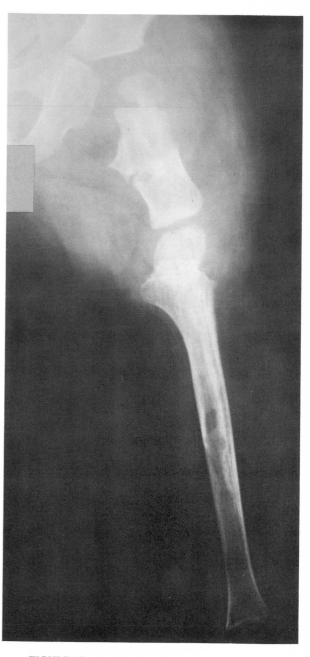

FIGURE 18   Solid fusion of knee at time of ankle disarticulation.

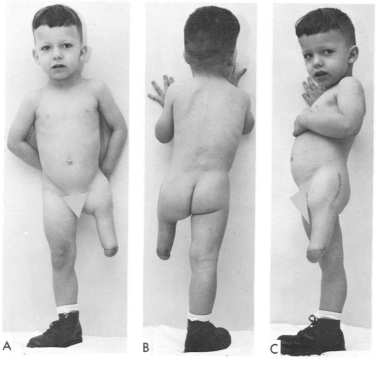

FIGURES 19-A, 19-B, and 19-C   Anterior, posterior, and lateral views of stump following surgery.

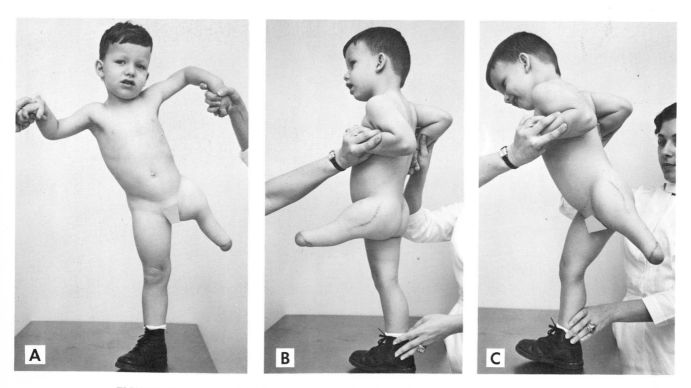

FIGURES 20-A, 20-B, and 20-C   Stump range of motion in flexion, abduction, and extension.

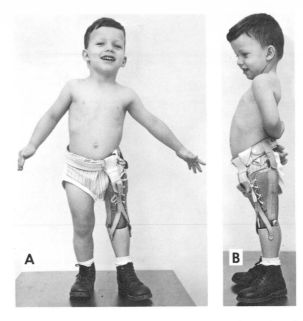

FIGURES 21-A and 21-B   Knee-disarticulation-type prosthesis provided following surgery.

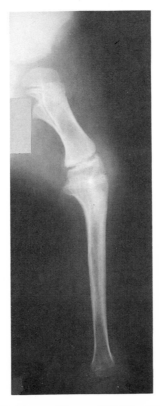

FIGURE 22   Epiphyses still open following surgical procedures.

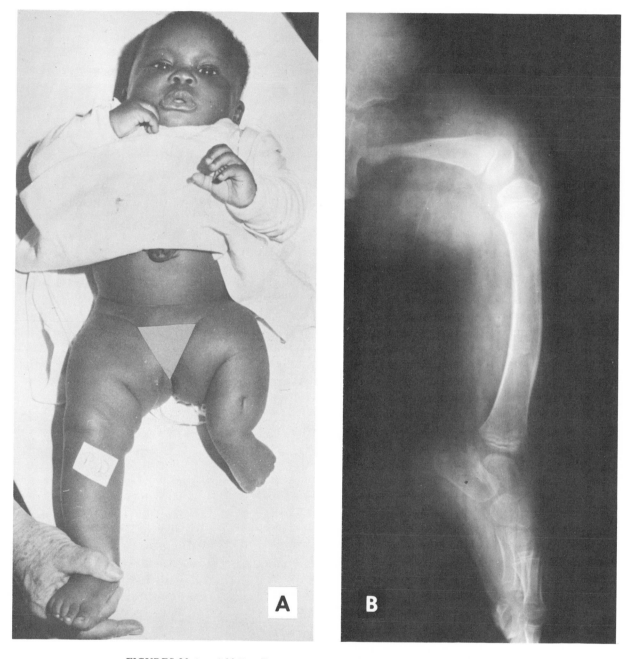

FIGURES 23-A and 23-B   External and x-ray views of patient's Type B PFFD.

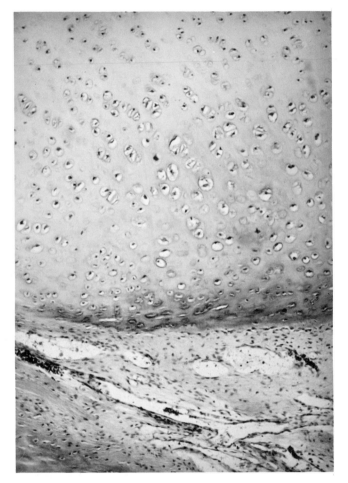

FIGURE 24   Viable cartilage taken from proximal femur.

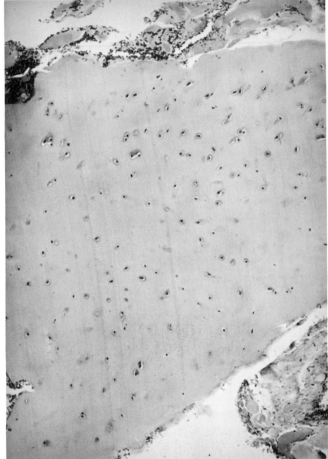

FIGURE 25   Section from the epiphysis of the femoral head.

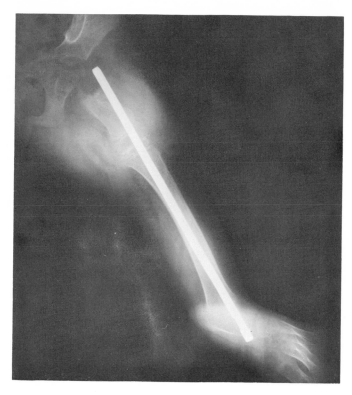

FIGURE 26   Thin spicular bone from femur to femoral head at
initial cast removal.

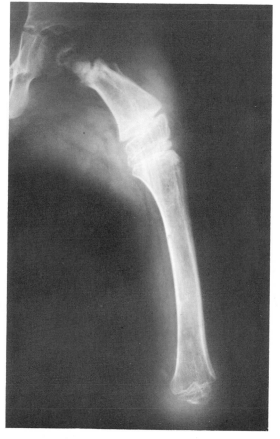

FIGURE 28   X-ray of stump following removal of
foot and intramedullary rod.

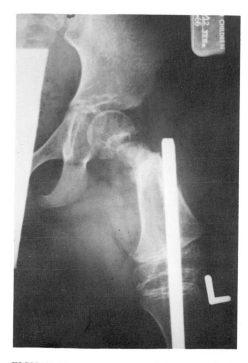

FIGURE 27   Hypertrophy of the bone spicule
ten months after surgery.

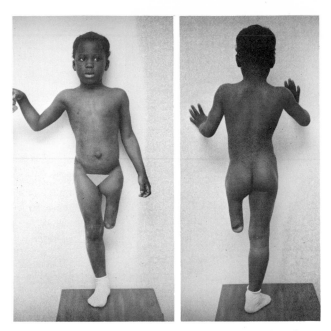

FIGURE 29   A stable hip eleven months after beginning of surgery.

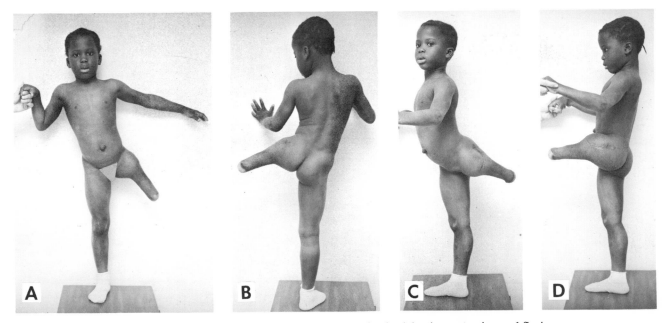

FIGURES 30-A through 30-D   Stump range of motion in abduction, extension, and flexion.

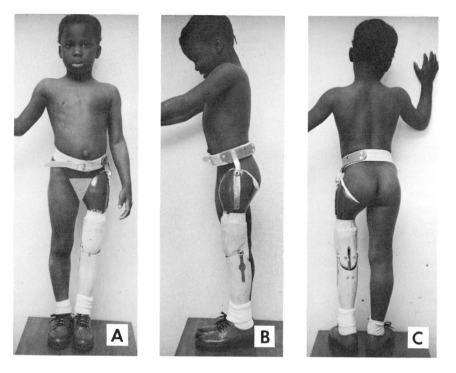

FIGURES 31-A, 31-B, and 31-C   Views of postoperative prosthesis.

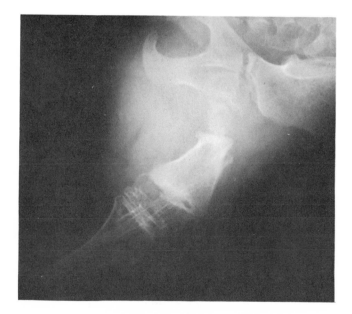

FIGURE 32   Line of translucency in femoral shaft 15 months after surgery.

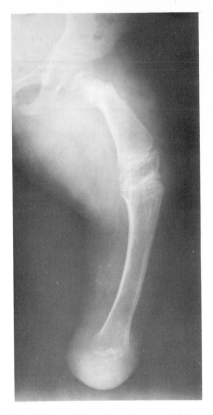

FIGURE 33   Closing of translucent zone eight months later.

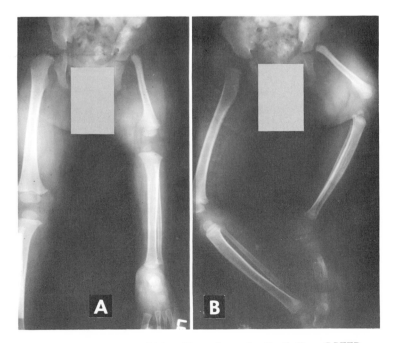

FIGURES 34-A and 34-B   X-ray views of patient's Type C PFFD.

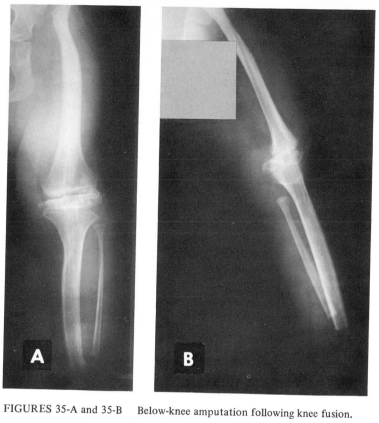

FIGURES 35-A and 35-B   Below-knee amputation following knee fusion.

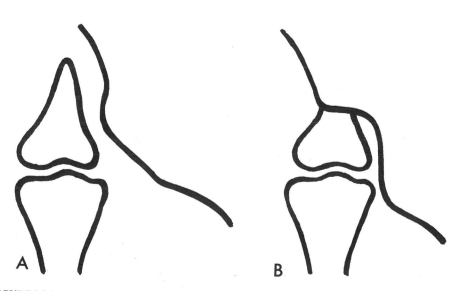

FIGURES 36-A and 36-B   Drawing of contemplated surgery in Type D PFFD to use knee as hip joint.

HARLAN C. AMSTUTZ, M.D.

The Morphology, Natural History, and Treatment of
PROXIMAL FEMORAL FOCAL DEFICIENCIES

Treatment of proximal femoral focal deficiencies (PFFD) depends largely on the anticipated growth and development of the affected limb. A classification scheme based on the morphological natural history of sixty-eight PFFD's in fifty-seven patients (Table 1) from the Hospital for Special Surgery, New York; the Royal National Orthopaedic Hospital, London; and the Hospital for Sick Children, London, has been developed to enable the surgeon to prognosticate accurately for the individual case of PFFD and to plan treatment at an early age (4, 5). Thirty-four extremities, followed serially without operative intervention for an average of 7.5 growth years with a range of two to fifteen (with seventeen the arbitrary maximum if the child was seen at birth), form the basis of the natural history study. The total length of comprehensive clinical and radiographic follow-up averaged 10.3 years for fifty-three patients, with four being under treatment for less than one year.

Proximal femoral focal deficiency is defined as the absence of some quality or characteristic of completeness of the proximal femur, including stunting or shortening of the entire femur. The broad terminology has been based on the classifications of Frantz and O'Rahilly (12), Hall et al. (13), and Burtch (9). A portion of the distal femur was always present even if only represented by a distal ossicle in the severest form of the anomaly. A coxa vara in addition to a shortening greater than that due to the varus alone is characteristic of even a mild degree of PFFD. Patients with developmental coxa vara (so-called congenital, infantile, cervical) are not included in the series (3).

The present PFFD classification scheme includes five morphologically distinct groups identifiable by roentgenograms at birth, with six subtypes nearly always defined by the fifth year. The diagrammatic representations illustrating the five major groups (Figure 1) typify the conditions for the approximate age range of one to two years; Figure 2 illustrates the subtypes at adolescence. At birth the differences between the groups are more subtle. Each group included a sufficient number of patients to establish a specific natural history. This classification plan includes congenital bowed femur with coxa vara (2), which has not always been included with the PFFD entities (1, 7, 8, 11, 15). The major PFFD groups are otherwise similar to Aitken's categories (1), but additional specificity for Types I and III has been added by subclassification (Figures 1 and 2).

Through the growth years a constant growth ratio of the normal to the abnormal limb was found in 87 percent of the PFFD extremities reviewed. An increase in inhibition of growth of three percent was noted in one patient, while a mean decrease of five percent with a range of three to ten was noted in seven. It is believed that technical mensuration errors in data, analyzed retrospectively, could have been responsible for these deviations. Proportionality of growth was demonstrated in every patient after five years of age. With careful attention to technical factors, precise prognostication will likely be possible as early as two years of age. By that age nearly all capital femoral epiphyses will have ossified, even though the ossification is later than normal.

Since the segments of the abnormal congenitally anomalous limb, as well as those of the normal limb, grow in length at a nearly proportionate rate for each PFFD type, precise length prognostication is possible (4). However, a methodology for accurate mensuration is essential, preferably using scanogram techniques and correcting for errors in projected length due to contractures. The limb-segment lengths are then plotted on a growth graph against skeletal age, and final lengths estimated.

A progressive coxa vara complicates mensuration and growth prediction. However, a growth ratio based on the

TABLE 1 Proximal Femoral Focal Deficiency Patients Reviewed

PFFD Type	Total Number of Extremities	Bilateral Symmetrical	Number of Extremities with Serial Follow-up	Mean Years Followed	Number of Extremities with Serial Follow-up for Length	Mean Growth Years Followed for Length	Age Range (Growth Years–17 Maximum)	Range Inhibition of Growth (%)	Mean Inhibition of Growth (%)
1A	13	–	13	8.3	9	7.6	2–15	26.8	16–38
1B	13	2	13	13.1	6	8.2	3–14	29.1	20–41
2	4	–	4	9.8	2	12.5	4–15	53.4	37–65
3	15[a]	–	14	13.8	10	5.9	3.3–15	50	35–60
4	9	–	9	9.3	5	6	2–12.6	64	36–80
5	14	5	10	7.2	2	12	10–14	87	79–95
	68	7[b]	63		34				

[a]1 patient Subtype A, 5 Subtype B, 1 Subtype C, 6 Subtype D, 3 not definitely classified prior to operation (1 probably Subtype B, 2 probably Subtype C).
[b]4 patients had bilateral asymmetrical PFFD's. Total patients included–57.

length of the femur measured from the lateral femoral condyle to the greater trochanter of the normal and abnormal limbs can be used for prognosticating the growth of the involved portion of the femur, since this segmental proportionality has also been verified.

Associated lower-leg anomalies accompanied 30 percent of Types I, II, and V and 50 percent of Types III and IV and added to or compensated for the shortening present.

MORPHOLOGY

PROXIMAL FEMORAL FOCAL DEFICIENCY TYPE V

In PFFD Type V, dysgenesis is so severe that none of the normal precursor hip-joint components, i.e., neither the capital femoral epiphysis nor the acetabulum, is present. Anatomically this condition was confirmed at operation by Mr. Lloyd-Roberts in one nine-month-old patient in this series. The hallmarks of this type are an iliac projection just above the usual acetabular anatomical site, present in eleven of fourteen hip regions, a spherical obturator foramen, and a "box-like" or square pelvis when the defect is bilateral. The severe deficiency extended to the middle and distal shaft in five patients with severe stunting and only a small bone segment that ossified late and represented the distal femoral epiphysis or femoral shaft (Figures 3-A and 3-B). Seven patients, including three affected bilaterally, for a total of 10 extremities, were followed for an average of 7.2 years. In four of these seven patients, a short femoral shaft developed but with severe proximal attenuation. Even though the proximal and distal femoral epiphyses appeared to be absent, the ossified portion of the femur continued to grow, although at a markedly inhibited rate.

Bilateral anomalies were present in six patients, five

symmetrically. On three of these we have no follow-up. One bilaterally involved patient also had vertebral anomalies and measured only 3 ft 3 in. in height at maturity. The ankle of the anomalous, unilateral, Type V extremity was positioned near the contralateral normal knee at maturity, permitting placement of a prosthetic functional "knee" center below the foot even if it were not amputated. All Type V patients had positive Trendelenberg and hip instability. The severity of the abductor lurch depended largely on the degree of external rotation and/or abduction contracture and the length of the thigh segment. The greater the external rotation and the longer the thigh segment, the more difficulty the patient has in shifting his center of gravity to provide stability, and the more marked the abductor lurch. One patient had a 90-deg external-rotation contracture so that knee extension and flexion appeared to represent hip "abduction–adduction." When the hip and knee joints are in close proximity, separation of "hip"- and knee-joint mobility and contractures is difficult. However, the true knee seemed to manifest excessive mobility and often developed crepitus in adolescence and adult life, especially when accompanied by significant external rotation and abduction contractures. Despite heavy activity, the patient on whom we have the longest follow-up remains symptom-free with some degree of flexion, abduction, and external-rotation contracture at the age of thirty-seven years. The degree of persisting contracture, especially in flexion, appears to reflect, at least partially, the method of prosthetic fitting with the patient "sitting" on his thigh. Flexion contractures averaged 35 deg in the unilateral patients and were more severe when the anomalies were bilaterally symmetrical. Operative findings have revealed considerable abnormality of musculature in these severe dysgeneses. However, the hypermobility and hip instability tend to lessen with age although the positive Trendelenberg remains.

PROXIMAL FEMORAL FOCAL DEFICIENCY TYPE IV

In Type IV the patient's dysgenesis is less severe with formed hip-joint components, although without an arthrogram this is sometimes difficult to ascertain with certainty at birth. An acetabulum and capital femoral epiphysis seemed to be present in all patients on whom roentgenograms were available during the first ten years of life and serve to differentiate Type IV from Type V (Figures 4-A and 4-B). Ossification of the capital femoral epiphysis is often delayed up to two and one-half years. Occasionally the greater trochanter will ossify separately, but ossification may be delayed up to four years. Characteristically the proximal end of the distal femoral shaft tapers sharply, almost to a point. This severe proximal attenuation differentiates Type IV from Type III and represents an unfavorable prognostic sign for naturally occurring ossification of the neck. Proximal migration of the tapered, often sclerotic, femoral shaft occurs because of weakness in the area of persisting pseudarthrosis. The acetabulum becomes dysplastic irrespective of the ossified capital femoral epiphysis. The iliac projection prominently noted in Type V was also present in two of nine Type IV patients. In one patient, a 90-deg external-rotation contracture was noted similar to that seen frequently in the unilateral Type V (Figure 5). Further passive external rotation of the hip was possible to 180 deg, although some of the rotation occurred at the knee.

The inhibition of growth in five unilateral patients averaged 64 percent and remained constant throughout growth for each individual patient but contractures and proximal migration increased the functional inhibition an additional 20 percent (*3*).

PROXIMAL FEMORAL FOCAL DEFICIENCY TYPE III

The infant with Type III PFFD appears clinically and roentgenographically similar to a mild Type IV in the first year, except that the ossified portion of the femoral shaft has a variable degree of proximal ossific bulbousness. The acetabulum is present, but ossification of the capital femoral epiphysis is often markedly delayed. The subsequent developmental course varied in the fifteen extremities included in this group, necessitating four subtypes (Figure 2), although the size and configuration of the proximal shaft are of diagnostic and prognostic importance.

Type III-A was characterized in one patient by eventual complete ossification and stability of the cervical and trochanteric regions (at the age of five years) without varus progression (Figures 6-A through 6-D). The stability exhibited by the initially wide deficient cervical area is unusual, and is associated with marked bulbousness without attenuation of the proximal femoral shaft.

The distinguishing features of PFFD Type III-B are

eventual complete ossification of the capital cervical trochanteric region, with marked varus progression that averaged 7.5 deg per year in four serially followed patients. Complete ossification was achieved by the age of six years for all four of these patients (Figures 7-A, 7-B, and 7-C). In three of the four patients the acetabulum became dysplastic in association with residual varus of 45 deg in two and 40 deg in one.

Spotty cervical ossification occurred in the single Type III-C patient with 115 deg of varus progression when followed to the age of eight years (Figures 8-A, 8-B, and 8-C). It is not likely that sufficient ossification will occur naturally to bridge the defect securely. This special subclassification is warranted when some ossification of a wide neck defect occurs, but the disturbance is so great that eventual complete stable bridging does not occur. This differentiation emphasizes the variability of ossification between III-A, III-B, and III-C types and has important treatment implications.

A wide persisting cervical pseudarthrosis characterizes Type III-D, although the capital femoral epiphysis, and frequently the trochanteric regions, ossifies. In the five patients of this type, three had marked proximal migration of the femoral shaft and progressive dysplasia of the acetabulum (Figures 9-A and 9-B).

Subgroup differentiation in infancy depends both on the qualitative and quantitative bulbousness of the proximal femoral shaft, but the length of the shaft has no prognostic significance. A large, broad, bulbously contoured, ossified proximal femoral shaft present in the first six months of life is likely to develop and morphologically become either Subtype III-A or Subtype III-B. On the other hand, some proximal attenuation of the femoral shaft, particularly if it persists into the third or fourth year, is likely to represent Type III-C or III-D. Careful follow-up is essential for proper subclassification, because a large bulb does not necessarily guarantee that the neck will ossify in some form.

Three other Type III PFFD patients had osteosynthesizing operations at an early age before precise subtyping was possible, although two seemed to be differentiating into Type III-C and the other into Type III-B.

The stability of the hip of the Type III PFFD varies and is dependent on such factors as neck-shaft continuity, varus, hip contractures, and femoral length. Considerable difficulty can be encountered in analyzing femoral growth in this group because of the varus progression and changeable hip-flexion contractures. In the present retrospective study, a proportionate inhibition of growth was found to remain constant in all of the Type III patients serially followed after the age of five years.

PROXIMAL FEMORAL FOCAL DEFICIENCY TYPE II

Type II PFFD is characterized by subtrochanteric pseudarthrosis and progressive varus, although the capitocervical area also has defective development, as manifested by delayed and irregular ossification. A higher incidence of the persisting subtrochanteric pseudarthrosis characteristic of Type II has been reported in patients where thalidomide had been an etiological factor (8). The morphology of the four patients in this group was somewhat heterogeneous, but the number of patients was insufficient to warrant subclassification. The classification of two short PFFD patients whose capital femoral epiphyses were ossified at one year and three months could not at that time be differentiated between Types II and III. A marked varus progression ensued in one, but the cervical region subsequently ossified with a persisting subtrochanteric defect characteristic of Type II (Figures 10-A, 10-B, and 10-C). The varus progression was not severe in the other patient and was perhaps modified by a drilling procedure performed at the age of two years. The subtrochanteric pseudarthrosis persisted to the age of ten and one-half years.

The subtrochanteric defect in a third patient simulated a pathological fracture through an ossific femoral attenuation. The area appeared to be healing with callus spontaneously when an osteosynthesizing procedure was performed at another hospital utilizing homogenous bone at three months of age. The area healed so that the femur is indistinguishable from Type I with a stable coxa vara and shaft bowing as described below (Figures 11-A through 11-D). A patient with a similar condition has been reported by Badger and Lambert (6). The possibility of traumatic insult at birth is real and had he not fractured he may well have been morphologically similar to one Type I patient with a subtrochanteric defect.

In the fourth patient the proximal portion of the femoral shaft was flattened with a superior tuft of irregular ossified material. His subtrochanteric pseudarthrosis apparently developed through this defective area with subsequent progressive varus. In addition to varus of the neck and subtrochanteric sites, two patients also had varus bowing of the shaft. Functionally these patients varied, but in general the hips were more stable than the more severe dysgeneses, although the Trendelenberg was positive.

PROXIMAL FEMORAL FOCAL DEFICIENCY TYPE I

Proximal femoral focal deficiency Type I, previously described as congenital bowed femur with coxa vara, is readily distinguishable from Types II and III by a stable, nonprogressive coxa vara and considerable femoral shaft bowing. Even in the first year, differentiation is possible because of the bowing of the femoral shaft and the concavity in the proximal–medial subtrochanteric area. There is medial femoral cortical sclerosis and often a laterally positioned beak.

Because of its early appearance, Type I PFFD has often been mistaken for congenital dislocation of the hip, since the shaft is laterally and proximally positioned (Figure 14-A). However, the shortening and bowing, which are often severe, point the way to the correct diagnosis (Figures 12-A, 12-B, and 12-C). In one patient the severe shaft bowing spontaneously diminished from 75 to 5 deg (Figures 12-B and 12-C), but characteristically the lesser trochanter failed to ossify.

The capital femoral epiphysis ossifies and is well centered in the acetabulum. However, ossification may be delayed. Follow-up films on all patients have revealed a stable coxa vara of between 90 and 115 deg except in two where neck–shaft angles of 120 and 125 deg were substantially reduced from the normal of 135 and 150 deg. However, a 30-deg midshaft varus produced a composite varus of 90 deg in the patient with the neck–shaft angle of 120 deg. It is important to emphasize that, to verify age changes of varus and bowing (5), serial roentgenograms need to be taken in two planes in a corresponding degree of rotation.

Eleven patients, two with bilateral involvement, were distinguished by the onset of progressive hip dysplasia which altered the prognosis with an early onset of degenerative arthritis and these have been categorized as Type I-B (Figures 13-A, 13-B, and 13-C). For some cases this differentiation was not obvious in early life. In seven patients between the ages of two and six years, dysplasia was noted on the first clinic visit. In two the capital femoral epiphysis was spherical in shape at the age of one and two years, respectively, only to become dysplastic by the time of subsequent follow-up visits between the ages of five and ten years. In ten of the eleven patients in this subtype, the capital femoral epiphysis became conical or bullet-shaped and the hip dysplasia progressed. In only one did the conical shape tend to become more spherical as the patient approached maturity.

All of the Type I-B patients had some abnormality of the combined capito-cervico-trochanteric epiphysis with a persisting (fetal) greater trochanteric-capital-femoral bridge in four (2), and a small epiphysis that ossified on the medial portion of an apparently broadened femoral neck in three. In one patient, marked irregularity of the capital femoral epiphysis was present in the first year of life, reminiscent of epiphyseal dysplasia. Three had irregular vertical epiphyseal lines and two had early acetabular dysplasia.

The neck–shaft angle of 95 deg for PFFD Type I-B was slightly less than the 106 deg of Type I-A, but the overlapping range of varus would indicate that this difference alone is not responsible for the onset of dysplasia in Type I-B. The shaft varus of PFFD Type I-B averaged 11 deg, compared with 14 deg for PFFD Type I-A. The exact etiology of dysplasia is, therefore, not apparent.

Inhibition of growth remained constant after all epiphyses were ossified in thirteen serially followed Type I-A and Type I-B patients, with the mean inhibition being 26.8 and 29.1 percent, respectively.

TREATMENT

The treatment of proximal femoral focal deficiencies must be based on a sound morphological analysis and an appreciation of the natural history according to classification type and subtype. The type and timing of operations to improve hip development and stability, and the management of leg-length inequality, depend on prognostication based on morphology and anticipated limb-length discrepancy. The indications for valgus osteotomy or osteosynthesis for progressive varus and abductor insufficiency must be based on a realistic appraisal of the functional improvement that can be achieved; that is, whether, if successful, the surgery will advance the patient to a morphological type with less anticipated functional impairment. Surgery, especially about the hip and the proximally deficient femur, has all too often resulted in an undesirable functional result. In this regard, our own experience dictates more often what not to do and, unfortunately, only occasionally what should be done.

PROXIMAL FEMORAL FOCAL DEFICIENCY TYPE I

The indications and advisability of performing a valgus osteotomy in Type I-A are not clear because of our inability to predict whether or not dysplasia of Type I-B will develop and if and when the varus of the femoral neck alone or possibly in association with retroversion may lead to a conical femoral head development.

Three Type I-A patients who have been followed to maturity with neck–shaft angles of 95, 90, and 105 deg, respectively, including one patient who was 66 years of age, had spherical femoral heads, so dysplasia does not necessarily develop with age.

Three Type I-A patients underwent valgus osteotomy. A 5-deg correction only was achieved in one patient on whom the osteotomy was performed through a subtrochanteric medial defect, with some delay in healing. The pre-existing retroversion was uncorrected, and at the age of twenty-four she has begun to experience a vague ache in her knee although no significant symptoms are thought to emanate from the hip. Two patients who had osteotomies at the age of four and thirteen, respectively, have been lost to follow-up. We do not have sufficient data to recommend or advise against a valgus osteotomy, since it is not certain that surgical restoration of a normal neck–shaft angle and anteversion will prevent the dysplasia and osteoarthritis that accompany Type I-B.

Since osseous continuity of the capito-cervico-trochanteric area will be established at an early age, and the coxa vara is not progressive, osteosynthesizing procedures are not indicated. An autogenous graft was inserted into one hip before precise morphological typing could be done, although, with the bowing and large bulbous proximal shaft, classification as Type I or III-A was logical (Figures 14-A through 14-D). In retrospect, further development would have established the type more precisely, and, if it had proven to be Type I, the operation probably could have been avoided.

When the femoral head dysplasia of Type I-B became evident with accompanying acetabular dysplasia, valgus osteotomies in five hips of four patients were accompanied by subluxation and further dysplasia with early onset of osteoarthritis. We would, therefore, advise against the use of valgus osteotomy alone when dysplasia is present, and it is merely a conjecture that, at the earliest sign of dysplasia, a Chiari pelvic osteotomy, or some other shelving procedure in combination with osteotomy, would prevent these changes.

PROXIMAL FEMORAL FOCAL DEFICIENCY TYPE II

An osteosynthesizing procedure is indicated in the presence of an increasing varus that results from pseudarthrosis in the subtrochanteric area. The timing of the operation is undoubtedly of considerable importance, and the surgery should be performed before the deformity becomes marked and secondary acetabular and femoral dysplasias develop. However, a sufficient amount of time should pass to allow for possible spontaneous ossification and union, even though a corrective valgus osteotomy may be required later. In this respect, decision for osteotomy and bone grafting in one patient might better have been postponed (Figures 11-A through 11-D). The varus might have diminished with growth.

PROXIMAL FEMORAL FOCAL DEFICIENCY TYPE III

Morphological subclassification is essential in Type III because of marked variability in prognosis from a remarkably similar infantile roentgenographic appearance. The rare Type III-A does not require an osteosynthesizing procedure or an osteotomy to prevent further varus. The same discussion about the indications for valgus osteotomy would apply to this subtype as to Type I-A.

The progressive varus of Type III-B is best treated by a valgus osteotomy. Possibly the operation should be delayed to allow maximum development of the capital femoral epiphysis. The ability to achieve full correction would not be compromised, since early closure of the capital femoral epiphysis is likely to occur with subsequent stunting. The operation should not be delayed, however, if symptoms, function, or impending dysplasia are apparent (Figures 15-A, 15-B, and 15-C). Technically, the interlocking osteotomy provides sufficient mechanical stability to obviate the need for internal fixation and a second operative procedure to remove the fixation. The procedure, as initially described for the progressive varus of the condition which is now preferably called developmental coxa vara, is applicable to this type (2). A strong spike of lateral cortex is fashioned in the distal fragment and mortised into a slot cut in the proximal fragment and controlled by a Steinmann pin (Figure 16).

For full correction or stability it may be necessary to transfix through the neck into the head. Mobilization of the fragments by subperiosteal stripping, abductor tenotomy, or detachment of abductor muscles may be necessary. If the mortise-and-tenon joint does not provide sufficient stability, percutaneous pin fixation of both fragments for six weeks is advisable. Anteroposterior and lateral roentgenograms to check the correction should be obtained prior to closure of the wound, and a minimum of ten weeks of immobilization in a double hip spica is absolutely essential.

Osteosynthesizing procedures for Type III-C present complex technical problems. The rudimentary disordered ossification in the femoral neck might be stimulated by a bridging graft combined with valgus osteotomy, although resection of all of the cartilaginous anlage would provide the most certain method of effecting union.

One osteosynthesizing procedure previously reported (*14*), when the subtyping differentiation between C and D was not yet clearly defined and involving a patient six months of age, led to a massive osseous bridge between the ilium and the greater trochanter which had required two subsequent operations for removal by the time of follow-up examination at five years and eight months of age. The cause of the new bone growth in this patient is not clear. Retrospectively, the degree of varus was not severe and perhaps the initial procedure should have been delayed to observe what further natural ossification would have occurred.

Contractures in this group are often severe, indicating considerable muscle abnormality. We have had no personal experience with casting or traction as advocated by Blauth (*8*). However, it is technically quite difficult to apply effective traction in a growing child with a short thigh segment. Even if the stress could be effectively relieved, subsequent weight-bearing and the effect of the abnormal muscle forces may lead to recurrence unless the other component abnormalities were stabilized by growth and development or operation.

A case involving excision of the head and neck and fibular transplant previously reported (*2*) subsequently sustained dislocation. This procedure is not recommended, since the fibular epiphysis does not continue to grow and thus would not contribute sufficient growth or morphology to be of value.

Osteosynthesizing procedures for Subtype D pose severe technical problems and will undoubtedly fail unless the cartilaginous neck anlage is excised and bone-to-bone contact is secured, as emphasized by Westin (*17*). This procedure necessitates a 180-deg valgus angle eliminating the femoral neck. These procedures will have to be carefully evaluated and the results compared to those obtained on a similar nonoperated group, since some patients often function surprisingly well without operation even though the hip is somewhat unstable and there is a positive Trendelenberg and abductor lurch.

PROXIMAL FEMORAL FOCAL DEFICIENCY TYPE IV

The severe stunting and marked anomalous musculature about the hip suggest difficulty in achieving a functional improvement even if an osteosynthesizing procedure were a technical success. Severe external rotation and abduction contractures, when present, create a most difficult problem because of marked instability. The person must awkwardly shift his weight far to the side for stability. The short thigh segment has little power in the normal flexion plane and knee extension and flexion appear to represent "hip abduction–adduction." The longer the thigh segment, the farther the weight must be shifted and the greater the abductor lurch. One patient, whose extremity could be externally rotated almost 180 deg passively, was fitted with the foot turned around as popularized by Van Nes, but because of the rotation, undue strain on the knee has occurred. We have had no experience in actually performing derotation osteotomies for this specific purpose, but have had the opportunity of following two performed at other hospitals. The theoretical advantage of converting the extremity to a functional below-knee amputation rather than one above the knee was not clinically apparent in these patients who required knee-extension assists despite the fact that they could flex and extend the "knee" by plantar and dorsiflexion of the ankle with good power. However, the hip was quite unstable in one and stiff in the other as a result of operative attempts to fuse the hip. Total evaluation was very difficult. For a girl the poor cosmetic effect of the Van Nes procedure may be unacceptable socially and psychologically. One male patient even developed severe psoriasis. The other patient required multiple operations, including two for complete derotation, two unsuccessful operations to fuse the hip, and a knee arthrodesis. The spontaneous tendency to derotate with growth, requiring further procedures, has been reported. Careful preoperative and postoperative functional evaluation of this procedure must be made to determine its ultimate value.

PROXIMAL FEMORAL FOCAL DEFICIENCY TYPE V

No hip surgery is indicated for proximal femoral focal deficiency Type V, since normal components are absent.

TREATMENT OF LEG-LENGTH INEQUALITY

All patients with proximal femoral focal deficiency, irrespective of type, present significant leg-length discrepancies, with the exception of the rare bilateral Type I (*4*). The predicted limb-segment discrepancy is determined by multiplying the percent inhibition of growth (difference between normal and abnormal length divided by normal times 100) by the anticipated normal limb-segment length. Serial scanograms are strongly recommended. The limb lengths are plotted on a Green and Anderson graph according to skeletal age. The predicted normal length is determined by transcribing the same spatial relationship of the growth curve to the mean-growth curve line at maturity.

The heights of the patient, obtained serially with sufficient block height to level the pelvis, are also plotted on a graph in order to prognosticate the ultimate height and determine the magnitude of the leg inequality, and to relate this to the child's estimated ultimate height. Recommendations for amputation must be individualized and based not only on the factors discussed above but also on projected intellectual capacity and personal, physical, and emotional needs. We have been impressed by the fact that the development of the child and his adjustment to life with a deformity are strongly dependent on the parents' understanding and attitudes. It is of particular benefit to be able to predict ultimate morphology and leg-length discrepancy and to prepare the parents at an early age for the ultimate treatment. We do not hesitate to perform an early amputation, particularly ankle disarticulation with immediate postsurgical prosthetic fitting and early weight-bearing, when this procedure is clearly the best form of treatment—as when the foot is abnormal with an associated paraxial fibular hemimelia and severe leg-length discrepancy. The amputations have been performed primarily to facilitate prosthetic fitting, since functional improvement in the active, growing child is not always apparent. In adolescence the improved cosmesis achieved through Syme's-type ankle amputations is of particular importance, especially to females, but we have been impressed by how well some of our patients have performed without amputation. Final evaluation of the merits of conversion amputations will require further time to compare all types of PFFD patients with varying degrees of leg-length discrepancies who have been treated by different methods and followed well into adult life. Ultimately we hope to be able to recommend treatment based on the individual physical, mental, and emotional makeup of the patient.

We have had little experience with the combined ankle-disarticulation and knee-arthrodesis procedures by which the patient is converted to a functional above-knee amputee with the ankle of the abnormal limb positioned either at the level of the normal knee or between the knee and ankle. We have functionally "arthrodesed" the patient's knee in extension within the prosthesis, resulting in a long-limb segment which has been attended with the usual problems of a fused knee and is tolerated best by short persons. One young PFFD Type III-D woman who is 5 ft 9 in. in height had a marked abductor lurch. Because of pain in the hip, knee, and back, presumably the result of the long extremity lever transmitting stress to the hip and back, a knee arthrodesis and a below-knee amputation were performed to provide her with a flexible prosthetic knee at the level of the normal knee.

Now that we are able to predict ultimate leg-length discrepancy (4), the surgical treatment could be performed at the appropriate age so that a femoral or tibial epiphysiodesis, or both, could be done at the time of knee arthrodesis and a Syme's-type end-bearing amputation rather than a below-knee amputation could be performed. A moderately severe proximal femoral focal deficiency in which it was predicted that the ankle would otherwise be opposite the middle of the contralateral normal leg would then mature with the prosthetic knee at the same level as the contralateral knee. This type of planning would result in a good end-bearing amputation stump of the ankle-disarticulation type as a definitive procedure. Recently we utilized this approach for a PFFD Type III-D with a 46 percent inhibition of femoral growth on whom the greater trochanter and capital femoral epiphysis were excised at eight months and the fibular head unsuccessfully transplanted into the femur. An ankle disarticulation and knee arthrodesis with distal femoral and proximal tibial epiphysiodesis were performed two weeks apart at the age of ten years and eleven months. The extremity was immobilized in a rigid plaster dressing and a pylon attached. The technique of knee arthrodesis and epiphysiodesis using a triangular template as a guide is illustrated (Figure 17).

The timing of the procedure was based on a growth analysis, using the Green and Anderson growth graph (Figure 18). By projection on the graph, the estimated length of the normal femur at maturity was 45.5 cm. Therefore, the arthrodesed femur and tibia of the abnormal limb should have a functional length about five centimeters less to allow space for the prosthetic knee-joint mechanism.

The anticipated length of the unaltered tibia, assuming that the growth pattern would continue along a line about equidistant between the mean and one standard deviation below it, was 37 cm. Transcribing the same spatial relationship of the patient's growth graph line for the tibia on the Green and Anderson graph for remaining growth of the proximal tibia, the length could be diminished 3.75 cm by epiphysiodesis at skeletal age 10 years plus 11 months. The net tibial length would then be approximately 32.2 cm.

The functional length of the abnormal femur was 15.2 cm at the time of operation (18.2 cm length minus 3 cm of proximal migration). The arthrodesis reduced the length an additional 4.3 cm so that the estimated combined length of the extremity will be 43.1 cm (15.2 − 4.3 + 32.2). Our growth studies indicate that less than anticipated growth may occur following ankle disarticulation, although more data must be accumulated to substantiate this indication. Therefore, it is possible that the limb segment may be shorter than predicted and allow enough space for the knee-joint mechanism below the long end-bearing Syme's-type stump at maturity and still have level knee centers. The technique of arthrodesis and the final result will merit further study.

When the thigh segment is longer and the leg-length

discrepancy is less, preservation of knee function and swing-phase control may be desirable despite the long prosthetic lower-limb segment which results. In such cases this approach might be preferable to knee fusion, and the choice would depend not only on the length of the thigh segment but also on the patient's height. Again a short person is functionally better able to accommodate a prosthetically lengthened lower-limb segment in many pursuits ranging from riding a bicycle to sitting in the theater. Undoubtedly, each PFFD patient must be analyzed individually, and the results of knee arthrodesis must be carefully followed.

As yet, there are no reports of the effect of increased stress on the abnormal hip resulting from knee arthrodesis. If fusion is performed, it is recommended that it be done with the knee in extension. Favorable reports indicate (*17*) that the hip contractures diminish in time. This result is most desirable for improvement of gait.

Knee arthrodesis of the externally rotated and abducted limb would increase the distance from the center of gravity as well as the amount of lateral shift and abductor lurch necessary to balance the unstable hip unless the contractures were corrected.

We have been gratified by the results obtained from fitting two bilaterally asymmetrical PFFD patients with double extension prostheses. The first patient had bilateral paraxial fibular hemimelias with two- and three-rayed feet in addition to PFFD Types III-B and III-D. Ankle disarticulations were performed with immediate postsurgical prosthetics fitting, and the patient's height was gradually increased from 3 ft 10 in. to 5 ft 2 in. to equal her span. At present she walks without support and has demonstrated remarkable improvement in social and intellectual achievement at school. Similar social improvement was noted in another patient who had a knee disarticulation for Type II PFFD and a contralateral Type I-A PFFD.

SUMMARY

Classification of proximal femoral focal deficiencies based on the natural history of specific types and subtypes is essential for prognostication of ultimate morphology. The deficient limb segment follows the rule of proportionality of growth in relation to the normal limb segment. Serial scanograms and determination of skeletal age enable the physician to predict ultimate leg-length discrepancy, plan treatment at an early age, and perform surgery at an appropriate age based on individual intellectual, personal, physical, social, and psychological needs.

The methods of treatment of the hip instability, contractures, and leg-length discrepancy associated with PFFD are described, and recommendations, where possible, have been made for specific types and subtypes. However, many forms of treatment which are now being applied to these challenging problems in this clinic and others around the world require continued careful analysis and follow-up. It is our hope that operative procedures for the PFFD patient will be based on a most careful morphological analysis and review of the experiences of many surgeons.

ACKNOWLEDGMENTS

The author would like to thank Mr. George Lloyd-Roberts, F.R.C.S., and Sir Herbert Seddon, and their respective hospital staffs, for allowing him to review the records of their patients.

BIBLIOGRAPHY

1. Aitken, G. T. Proximal femoral focal deficiency. Personal communication.
2. Amstutz, H. C., and P. D. Wilson, Jr. Dysgenesis of the proximal femur (coxa vara) and its surgical management. J. Bone Joint Surg. 44A(1):1–24, 1962.
3. Amstutz, H. C. Developmental coxa vara—a distinct entity. To be published.
4. Amstutz, H. C. Prognostication of length for congenital anomalies of the lower limbs. To be published.
5. Amstutz, H. C. The natural history and classification of congenital anomalies of the femur. To be published.
6. Badger, V. M., and C. N. Lambert. Differential diagnosis of an apparent proximal focal femoral deficiency. ICIB V(1):3–9, October 1965.
7. Bevan-Thomas, W. H., and E. A. Millar. A review of proximal femoral focal deficiencies. J. Bone Joint Surg. 49A(7):1376–1388, 1967.
8. Blauth, W. Der Kongenitale Femurdefekt. Stuttgart: Ferdinand Enke Verlag, 1967.
9. Burtch, Robert L. Nomenclature for congenital skeletal limb deficiencies: A revision of the Frantz and O'Rahilly classification. Artif. Limbs 10(1):24–35, 1966.
10. Dunn, A. W., and G. E. Aponte. Congenital bowing of the tibia and femur—Case report with autopsy findings. J. Bone Joint Surg. 44A(4):737–740, 1962.
11. Fock, G., and M. Sulaman. Congenital short femur. Acta Orthoped. Scand. 37:294–300, 1965.
12. Frantz, C. H., and R. O'Rahilly. Congenital skeletal limb deficiencies. J. Bone Joint Surg. 43A(8):1202–1224, 1961.
13. Hall, C. B., M. B. Brooks, and J. F. Dennis. Congenital skeletal deficiencies of the extremities. J.A.M.A. 181:590–599, 1962.
14. Lloyd-Roberts, G. C., and K. H. Stone. Congenital hypoplasia of the upper femur. J. Bone Joint Surg. 45B(3):557–560, 1963.
15. Shands, A. R., Jr., and G. D. MacEwen. Congenital anomalies of the femur. Acta Orthoped. Scand. 32:307–314, 1962.
16. Van Nes, C. P. Rotation-plasty for congenital defects of the femur. J. Bone Joint Surg. 32B:12–16, 1950.
17. Westin, W. Proximal femoral focal deficiency. Personal communication.

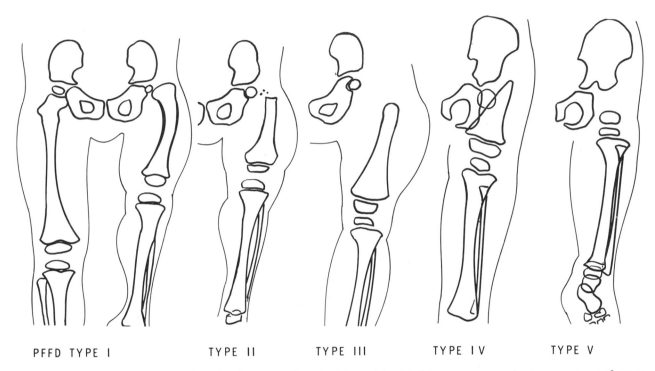

PFFD TYPE I   TYPE II   TYPE III   TYPE IV   TYPE V

FIGURE 1   Diagrammatic representation of major types of proximal femoral focal deficiency, corresponding to an age range of one to two years.

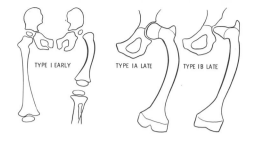

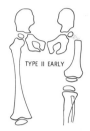
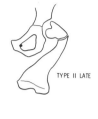

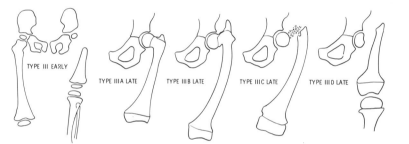

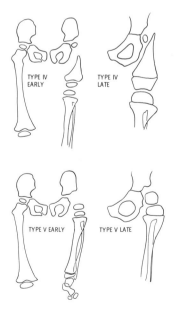

FIGURE 2   PFFD types and subtypes. Diagrammatic representation of undifferentiated types at approximate age of one year (left) and the developmental variations in adolescence (right).

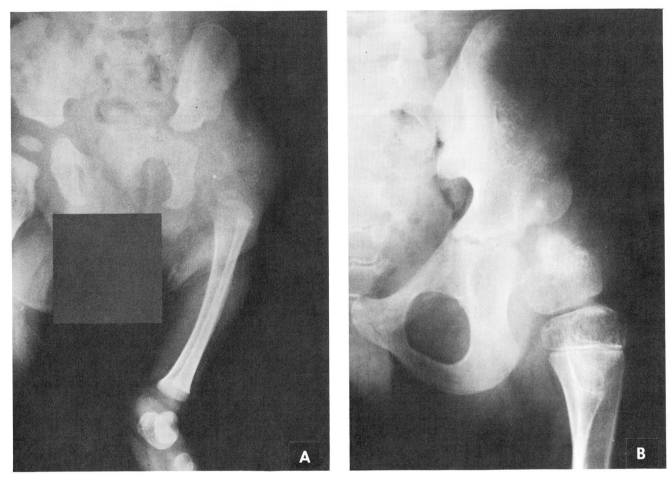

FIGURE 3-A   L.C., PFFD Type V—age one year. Absent acetabulum with iliac projection. Note external rotation of femur.
FIGURE 3-B   At age 10 years. Ossified distal femoral bone segment. Foot opposite normal ankle.

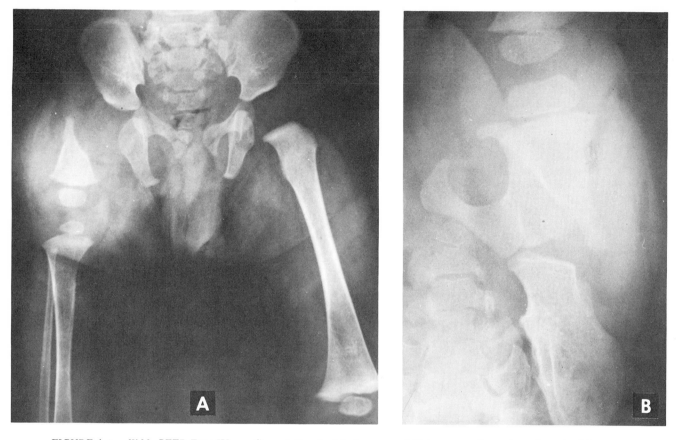

FIGURE 4-A   W.M., PFFD Type IV—age five months. Acetabulum present. Note severe attenuation of proximal femur.
FIGURE 4-B   W. M.—age two years. Ossification of capital femoral epiphysis. Note proximal migration.

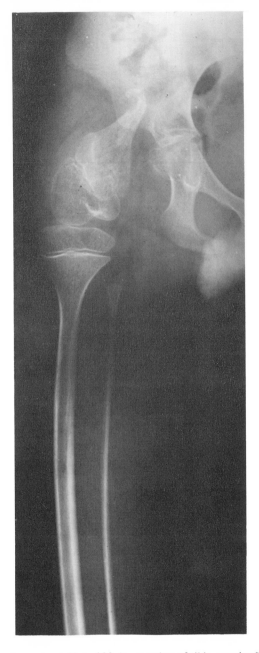

FIGURE 5   A.T., PFFD Type IV—age eleven years. Note 180-deg rotation of tibia, proximally tapered femoral shaft, ossified capital femoral epiphysis, and iliac projection.

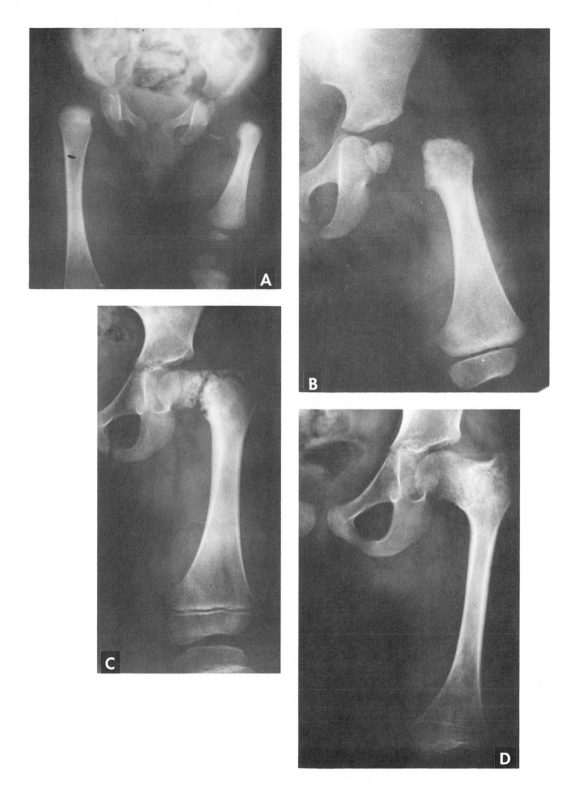

FIGURE 6-A   M.B., PFFD Type III-A—age fifteen months. Laterally placed femoral shaft with wide nonossified cervical region. Note
    large bulb of proximal femoral shaft.
FIGURE 6-B   Age two years and three months. Ossification of capital femoral epiphysis.
FIGURE 6-C   Age five years and four months. Ossification of cervical region without varus progression.
FIGURE 6-D   Age six years and ten months. Stable healed coxa vara with apparent early closure of capital femoral epiphysis.

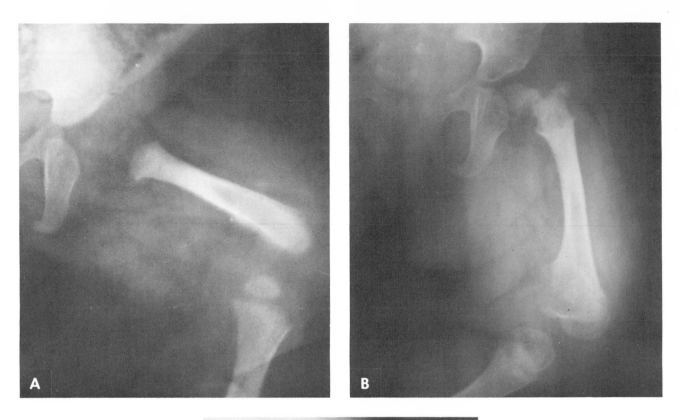

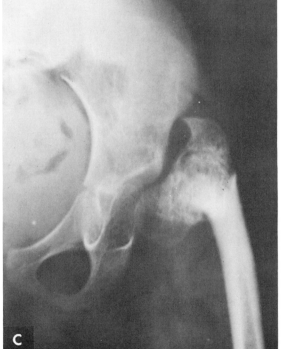

FIGURE 7-A   L.B., PFFD Type III-B—age four months. Note broad bulbous ossified portion of proximal femoral shaft.
FIGURE 7-B   Age two years and seven months. Ossification of the cervical region. The capital femoral epiphysis ossified at eight months.
FIGURE 7-C   Age six years. Note varus progression and persistence of fetal bridge between capital femoral and greater trochanteric epiphyses.

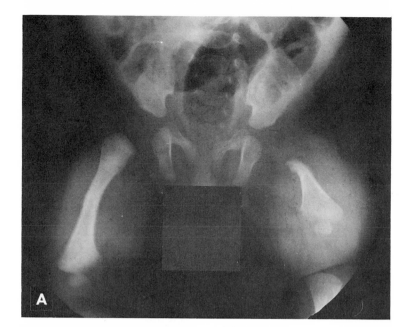

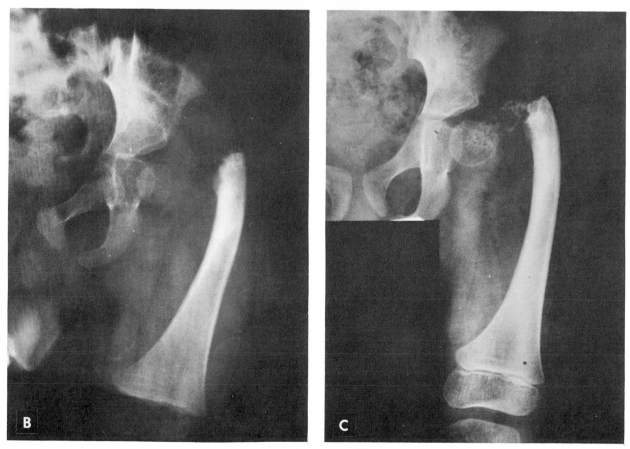

FIGURE 8-A   R.H., PFFD Type III-C—age two months. Very small bulb of proximally attenuated femoral shaft. Note contralateral short femur without coxa vara.

FIGURE 8-B   Age two years and nine months. Note proximal femoral migration.

FIGURE 8-C   Age seven years. Spotty cervical ossification. Further varus progression.

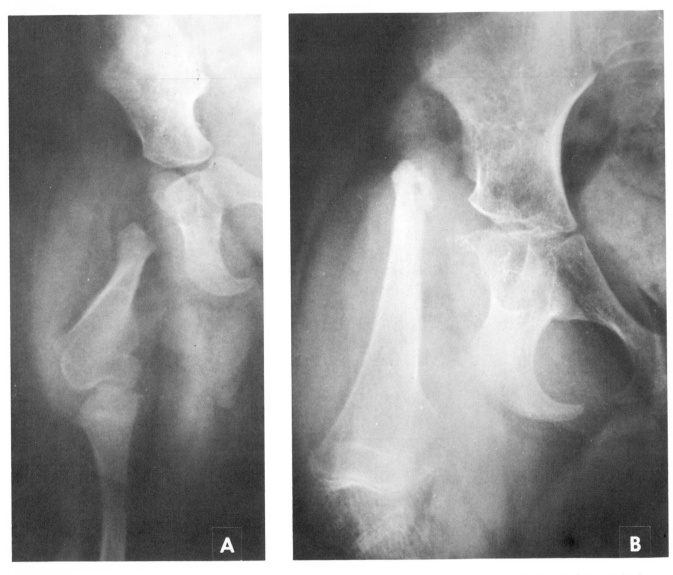

FIGURE 9-A   L.B., PFFD Type III-D—age nine months. Ossified capital femoral epiphysis and moderate bulbousness of the proximal
    femoral shaft.
FIGURE 9-B   Age six years. Proximal migration without ossification of cervical region.

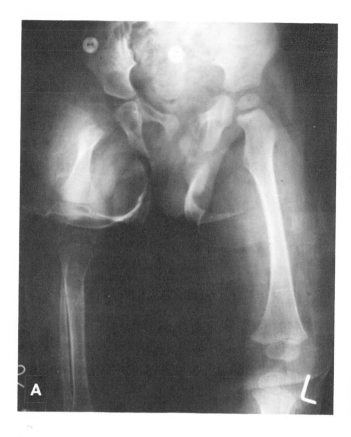

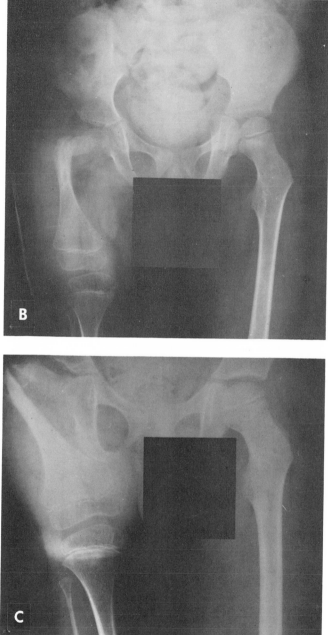

FIGURE 10-A   M.H., PFFD Type II–age one year and three months. Note broad proximal bulb, ossified capital femoral epiphysis, absent cervical ossification.

FIGURE 10-B   Six years and four months. Subtrochanteric pseudarthrosis with varus. Cervical ossification without varus.

FIGURE 10-C   Eight years and two months. Further varus progression. Note greater trochanteric ossification.

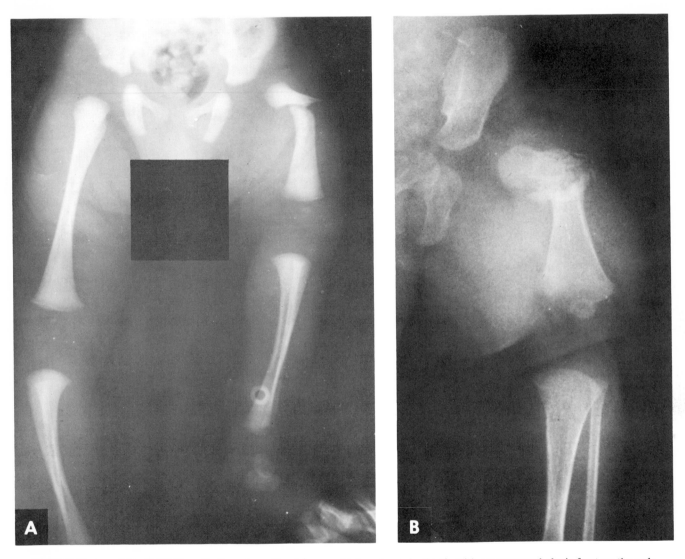

FIGURE 11-A   B.V., PFFD Type II—three days. Short femur with broad proximal bulb with apparent pathologic fracture through attenuated portion and varus angulation.

FIGURE 11-B   Three months. Preoperative. Note callus formation and early union in varus.

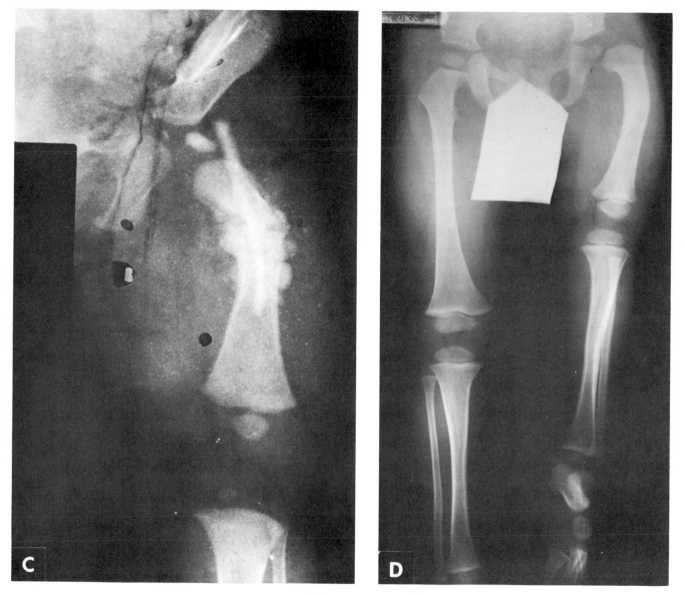

FIGURE 11-C   Postoperative—osteotomy and homogenous bone grafting.
FIGURE 11-D   Age one year and nine months. Stable coxa vara now similar to Type I.

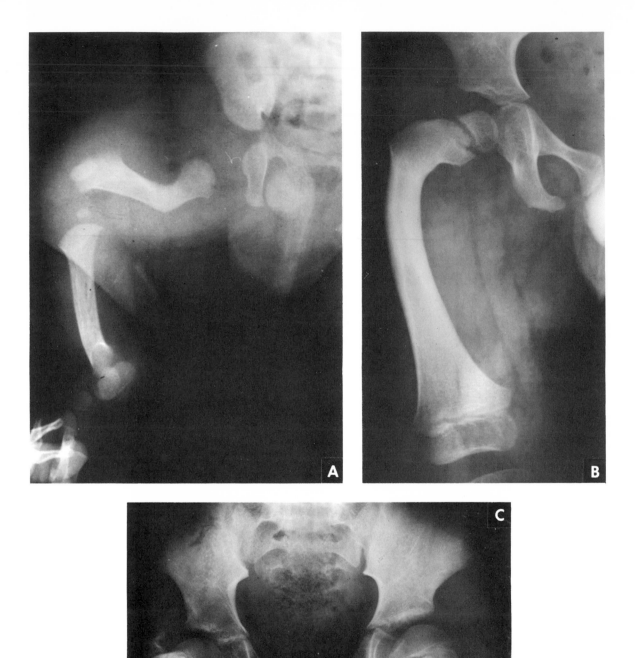

FIGURE 12-A   G.D., PFFD Type I-A—three months. Bulbous proximal femur with medial subtrochanteric concavity, severe bowing of approximately 75 deg.

FIGURE 12-B   Age four and a half years. Marked spontaneous diminution of shaft varus.

FIGURE 12-C   Residual shaft varus 5 deg. Neck–shaft angle 105 deg, without varus progression. Composite neck and shaft varus 100 deg.

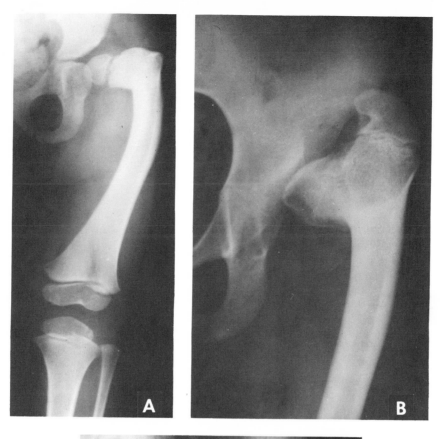

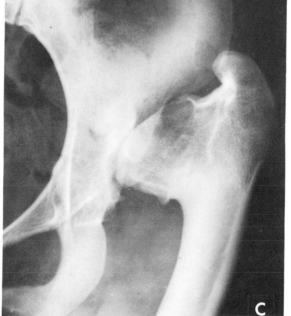

FIGURE 13-A   B.N., PFFD Type I-B—age two years. Round capital femoral epiphysis. Neck–shaft angle 90 deg. Twenty-five deg of
    femoral shaft varus.

FIGURE 13-B   Age ten and one-half years. Stable coxa vara. Note conical head, dysplastic acetabulum, and greater trochanteric overgrowth.

FIGURE 13-C   Age fifteen and one-half years. Early onset of secondary osteoarthritis.

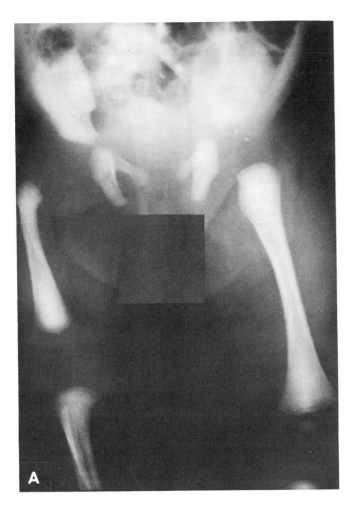

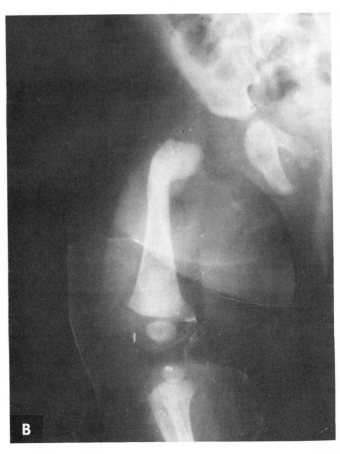

FIGURE 14-A   S.S., PFFD Type I—age one week. Laterally and proximally positioned femoral shaft.
FIGURE 14-B   Age six months. Preoperative.

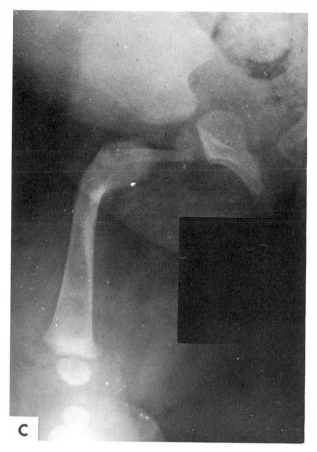

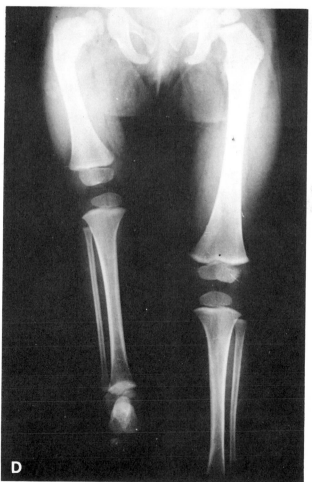

FIGURE 14-C   Postoperative. Autogenous graft.

FIGURE 14-D   Age one year and nine months. Additional intervening abduction osteotomy and removal of implant operations performed. Some asymmetry of capital femoral epiphysis and residual varus.

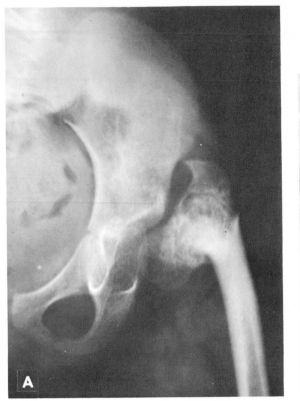

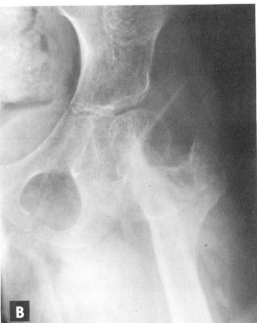

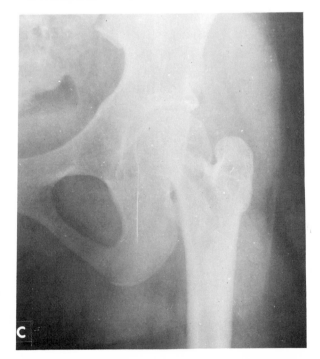

FIGURE 15-A   L.B., PFFD Type III-B—age six years. Neck–shaft angle (NSA) 45 deg.
FIGURE 15-B   Age six and one-half years. Postoperative interlocking osteotomy. NSA 180 deg.
FIGURE 15-C   Age twelve years. NSA 165 deg. Relatively concentric head and acetabulum.

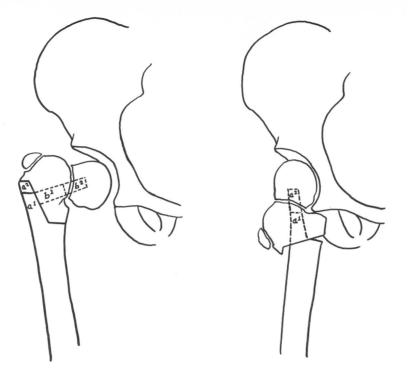

FIGURE 16   Drawing of the intertrochanteric interlocking osteotomy. The length of the lateral spike shaft (a^1 and a^2) and depth of the neck mortise (b^1 and b^2) may be varied, depending on the correction angle and the desirability of crossing the epiphyseal plate with the spike.

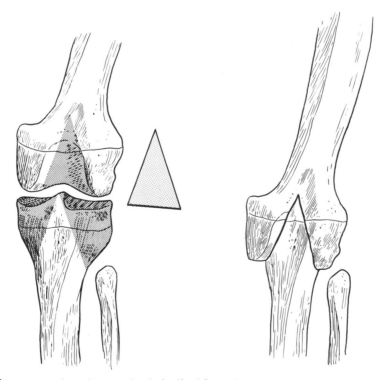

FIGURE 17   Diagrammatic representation of knee arthrodesis, distal femoral and proximal tibial epiphysiodesis. Note the template used to facilitate removal of bone wedges.

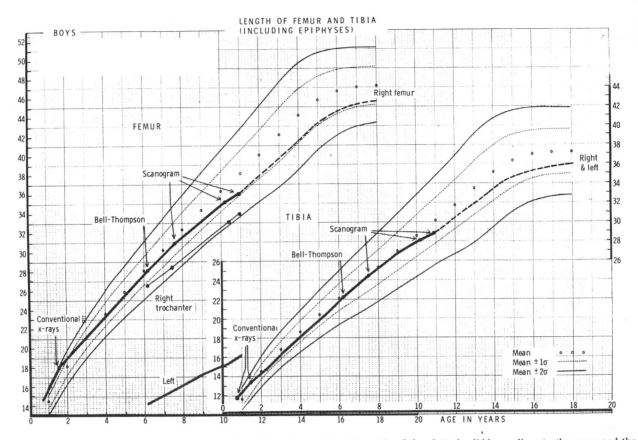

FIGURE 18   Femoral and tibial growth graph for R.R. Note the spatial relationship of the plotted solid heavy lines to the mean and the one and two standard deviation lines. The estimated growth for the normal femur and tibia are indicated by the heavy dashed line. (Graph adapted from Green, W. T., and M. Anderson. Growth and predictions of growth in lower extremities. J. Bone Joint Surg. 45A:1–14, 1963.)

JOHN E. HALL, M.D., F.R.C.S.(C)
DIETRICH BOCHMANN, C.P.O.(C)

The Surgical and Prosthetic Management of
PROXIMAL FEMORAL FOCAL DEFICIENCY

Proximal femoral focal deficiency is a complex deformity which can affect one or both lower extremities in varying degrees. Other congenital anomalies are frequently associated with the condition. There is no single approach to treatment that can be applied to every patient. Each must be assessed individually, as the problem may be functional in one child, and merely a matter of cosmesis in another. When treating patients with this condition, one must be prepared to use all modalities, including surgery and special prosthetic fitting, if optimal appearance and function are to be provided for these patients.

When both lower extremities are involved the condition generally tends to be more severe, and one of the major difficulties encountered is the extreme loss of height. This problem of short stature is accentuated by the fact that there is usually a severe hip-flexion deformity with the short femur lying almost parallel to the ground when the child is standing. These children have a waddling-type gait, but it is usually very effective, although their bodies are close to the ground. The prime difficulty is one of cosmesis and the physician is often forced into a position where he must choose between appearance and function. By the use of braces which keep the thigh segment and the shank in line, it is possible to add considerable height to the child, but this treatment results in considerably decreased agility (Figures 1-A and 1-B). Even more height can be added by the use of extension prostheses which keep the knees fairly straight and add height by a segment below the feet, either with or without a knee joint. Through the use of these prosthetic extensions the child can be brought up to normal height, but activities are greatly curtailed, and the final choice of management procedures in this type of patient will often lie with the child himself and with the parents.

When only one leg is affected, the main problem is one of discrepancy in length of the legs, although hip instability can be an added problem, depending on the configuration of the upper end of the femur (1). In this group of children, provision of a prosthesis is usually indicated. Whether or not any type of surgical intervention is warranted will depend on the amount of leg-length discrepancy and the actual configuration of the hip and ankle joints.

BILATERAL PROXIMAL FEMORAL FOCAL DEFICIENCY

Five children with severe degrees of this deformity are being managed through the Amputee Clinic of the Ontario Crippled Children's Centre. An attempt has been made to obtain a balance between appearance and function, recognizing that increasing the height of these children to that of their peers may be of little benefit if they are not mobile enough to play or even walk with them. Before the age of four they are probably best left alone, but as school age approaches both the family and the child may wish to try some type of appliance which will make the child less obviously different from his or her playmates.

Figures 2-A through 2-G and 3-A through 3-H illustrate types of devices that have been used. These devices range from simple braces which hold the knees straight to articulated extension prostheses having knee joints and proper feet.

When bilateral proximal femoral focal deficiency is combined with a distal anomaly, such as a fibular hemimelia and a deformed foot, consideration may then be given to surgical conversion (perhaps by a Syme's-type operation) to make fitting easier and more efficient. This type of approach should only be used, however, for a child whose deformities do not allow him useful ambulation without his prostheses. As stressed above, no prosthesis can replace the agility these children possess with their short extremities, providing their feet are plantigrade. Even if extension prostheses are provided, children will usually remove them within the confines of their own home, and nothing should be done surgically to deprive them of this possibility.

Figures 4-A through 4-E depict a young girl with bilateral PFFD with which were associated hypoplastic tibiae and severe clubfeet (partially corrected). Nonprosthetic ambulation was impossible and the malformed feet made prosthetic fitting difficult. Following bilateral Syme's amputations, prosthetic fitting was simpler and more cosmetic, while function without the prostheses was unaffected.

Figures 5-A and 5-B illustrate the treatment of a boy with a unilateral PFFD and an amelia on the opposite side. Independent ambulation was attained with a Canadian hip-disarticulation prosthesis, extension brace, and special crutches.

In all five of the patients illustrated, the hip deformity was a severe one, and no surgical reconstruction of the hip joint was undertaken. When devices were provided, the hip instability was managed by an ischial shelf on the prostheses.

As the children in this group approach the end of their growth years, consideration should be given to the performance of a knee arthrodesis to overcome the hip-flexion deformity, and to overcome some of the height deficit which is caused by the squatting stature associated with the PFFD.

UNILATERAL PROXIMAL FEMORAL FOCAL DEFICIENCY

A knowledge of the anticipated final leg-length discrepancy is probably the best guide to the type of management that will be most appropriate for these children. In this regard the work of Amstutz and Wilson (2) on predictive measures is most valuable. In reviewing a large number of cases, they have observed that there is a constant percentage of retardation of growth on the involved side, so that a knowledge of the actual amount of discrepancy compared to the length of the normal limb will permit calculation of an approximate amount of discrepancy one is likely to encounter at the completion of growth.

By the time a child is approximately three years of age, one should be in a position to tell how much of a problem this difference in leg length is likely to be, and plan a rational form of treatment based on this knowledge.

If the predicted difference is 3 in. or less, then the discrepancy can be best managed by the standard methods of leg equalization, including lifts or raises on shoes, epiphyseal arrest or leg shortening on the long side, and attempts at

growth stimulation or mechanical lengthening on the involved side. Since the deformity is relatively mild in this group of patients, the foot is usually a good one and the hip is not too badly involved. Hence, a reasonable result can be anticipated without the need for prosthetic management.

If the final discrepancy is expected to be in excess of 5 in., then this child will surely present a prosthetic problem. For children in this group, one will have to decide at some time whether or not some type of surgical conversion will be worthwhile. When the discrepancy is likely to be between 3 and 5 in., then, as in many other areas of orthopedic surgery, one is dealing with a borderline situation, and decisions must be based on surgical and prosthetic judgment and discussion of the problem with the parents and with the child, if he is old enough to participate.

Prosthetic management may entail as small an item as a simple shoe raise, which is usually all that is necessary for the mild case from the latter part of the first year through the second year of life. Other types of raises varying from the O'Connor boot to the simple extension prosthesis may be used according to the age and condition of the child.

Figures 6-A and 6-B show a young boy with a typical unilateral PFFD without associated defects. At the age of 18 months he was fitted with an O'Connor boot, and raises were added to the sole as he grew older. Eventually, he was provided with a simple plastic laminate extension prosthesis (Figure 6-C). Figure 7 depicts another child fitted with an O'Connor boot.

A more pronounced leg-length discrepancy in a young girl is shown in Figures 8-A and 8-B. She was wearing an extension brace (Figures 8-C and 8-D) when first seen at the clinic.

Another young boy with considerable leg-length discrepancy was fitted with an extension prosthesis without knee joints at a very early age (Figures 9-A, 9-B, and 9-C). Still another, whose anomalous right foot was at the level of the normal left knee, was provided with knee joints very early in his prosthetics career (Figures 10-A and 10-B).

In older children whose parents reject surgical intervention, a reasonably satisfactory extension prosthesis can be provided (Figures 11-A and 11-B). However, when parental and patient agreement can be secured, removal of the foot and fitting with a knee-disarticulation-type prosthesis is perhaps an even more satisfactory procedure for such patients (Figures 12-A and 12-B).

ROTATION OSTEOTOMY

There are many types of surgical management programs which may be used for the group of patients with 5 in. or more of leg-length discrepancy, including removal of the foot and then fitting the patient as a knee-disarticulation amputee. It is in this group that one may also consider a surgical rotation of the limb through 180 deg, so that the ankle joint can be used to operate the knee joint of a prosthesis.

This principle of rotating the foot was first used by Borggreve in 1930 (4) in a patient with a short femur secondary to an infection. Rotation was performed through the shaft of the femur.

In 1950, Van Nes described three cases in which he had rotated congenitally short lower extremities, so that the ankle joint could be used to give active control of the knee joint (5). The ages of these patients were one, nine, and fifteen years, respectively. In the youngest patient, part of the rotation was performed through a pseudarthrosis at the upper end of the femur, and the rotation was completed through a knee arthrodesis. In the nine-year-old, part of the rotation was performed through a knee arthrodesis and the remainder was subsequently obtained through a tibial rotation osteotomy. In the third child, all of the rotation was performed through a knee arthrodesis with sufficient resection of the lower end of the femur and the lower end of the tibia to effect the rotation safely. In each of these patients the final level of the ankle joint approximated the level of the opposite knee joint, and the patients learned to control the knee of the prosthesis very effectively.

There is little to add to the original description of this procedure, except that the main problem is a prosthetic, not a surgical, one. The surgical procedures are not complicated, but the prosthetics fitting is difficult, and it requires the services of a skilled prosthetist, particularly in the design of the foot socket and knee joint.

When considering whether or not to advise this type of procedure, one must realize that it has both advantages and disadvantages. The extension prosthesis, while giving quite an effective gait, is an awkward device, which will not bend at the knee either during walking or sitting. The principal advantage of the rotation type of osteotomy is that with it the child can obtain some control of the prosthetic knee unit and can bend his or her knee on sitting, kneeling, and bicycle riding.

One disadvantage of the rotation osteotomy is that the rotated foot presents a rather strange appearance when the prosthesis is off, and since one usually shortens the limb while it is being rotated, the patient's function without the prosthesis is typically diminished. The child is then usually put into a position where it is necessary for him to wear his prosthesis full time after the rotation has been accomplished. The appearance of the stump can be improved by removal of all of the toes, but this gain must be balanced by the loss of power in the stump, and also a loss of position sense and the feeling the child has that he can grip his prosthetic socket with his toes. The argument in favor of removing the toes is that fitting becomes slightly easier, since the stump has a rounded contour.

A further problem which may arise if the child has not

completed his growth by the time of his rotation is that the twisted musculature will tend to gradually derotate the leg. Of the nine patients who have had this procedure performed before the age of 12 years, four have already required repeat rotation osteotomies within three years of the original procedure, and the remainder will probably require rerotation also (Figures 13 and 14).

The necessity of repeated osteotomy could be avoided by waiting until the end of growth, but it may well be that the advantage of learning to use the ankle as a knee joint at an early age outweighs the relatively minor surgery involved, even if it has to be repeated once or twice before the end of the growth years.

The rotation can be accomplished at almost any level in the leg, and the final position, both with regard to rotation and level of the knee joint, is usually obtained by arthrodesis of the knee. This procedure is also valuable in overcoming the hip-flexion deformity found in the more severe types of hip involvement.

Nineteen patients with unilateral proximal femoral focal deficiencies are being followed at the Amputee Clinic at the Ontario Crippled Children's Centre, and the nine patients who were selected for rotation osteotomy were those deemed to have the best chance of benefiting from this procedure, and whose parents agreed to have it performed.

Figures 15-A through 15-D show the anatomical and prosthetic status of a young boy before and after rotation osteotomy.

Figures 16-A through 16-G illustrate another case of rotation osteotomy in which the toes were removed to improve the appearance of the stump. The excellent gait achieved by this child is shown in a series of frames from her film clip (Figure 16-H).

PROSTHETIC FITTING

As previously mentioned, one of the decisive factors determining whether or not a rotation osteotomy will be successful is the level of prosthetic management. A description of procedures follows:

CASTING

When the cast of a Van Nes rotation-osteotomy stump is being taken, two areas of weight-bearing are defined—the ischium and the heel. Once the full-length stump sock (cotton stockinette stitched in a half-moon shape at one end) is applied, the top of the sock is held firmly by an assistant. The plaster-of-Paris wrapping begins around the ischium and ilium and extends distally about three inches and proximally two inches to the ischial tuberosity. At this point no further casting should be done until this section has been molded into a quadrilateral shape. The technique of shaping by hand can give satisfactory results, or a casting device* can be used. While the assistant holds this quadrilateral socket cast against the ischium to ensure constant seating, the knee flexion which is present in many cases is now corrected.

With the knee held in its fullest extension, casting is continued distally from the shaped proximal section to just above the ankle and then is taken back to connect again with the quadrilateral-shaped section above. The assistant now moves to hold the foot in maximum plantar flexion for completion of the wrapping. A shelf, similar to the PTB shelf, is shaped on the plantar side of the calcaneus by simply applying pressure with the index finger on the long plantar ligament. Finally, plumb lines should be marked for reference on the lateral and anterior surfaces with the patient standing. When filling the cast to make the male mold, the holding pipe should be set parallel to these lines. This is necessary so that the holding pipe can be used as a reference line to transfer the plumb lines to the laminated socket later. The distance from the distal end of the cast to the floor should also be determined and the space available for filler blocks and/or the alignment jig[†] and the SACH foot noted. This is done by placing blocks under the cast, while the patient is still standing.

The male model is modified as required. Areas are built up where pressure relief is desired. Reliefs for the toes and ankle and other bony prominences are particularly important.

FABRICATION OF SOCKET

Lamination procedures require the use of one layer of Dacron felt and three layers of nylon stockinette. Polyester resin[‡] in a mixture of 70 percent flexible (P43) and 30 percent rigid (P13) is used. Suction, by means of a vacuum pump, is strongly recommended because of undercut areas where the laminate has to be drawn into the shape of the cast.

ALIGNMENT

Plumb lines on the cast should be transferred to the laminate using the holding pipe as a reference. The socket should be set into a filler block in accordance with these plumb lines. If space permits, a BK adjustable pylon is used; if the length is too short to accommodate an adjustable unit, filler blocks are used.

*VAPC Casting Stand, available from U.S. Manufacturing Co., Glendale, Calif.
†Berkeley Adjustable Below-Knee Jig, available through A. J. Hosmer Corp., Campbell, Calif.
‡Polyester Resins, available through Rohm & Haas Company of Canada Ltd., West Hill, Ont.

The axis of the mechanical knee joints is located 3/8 in. distal to the malleolus on the lateral aspect of the stump. The knee joints are aligned and their position marked on the socket.

The thigh socket can now be separated from the foot socket and trimmed. Trim-line details are shown in Figure 17.

The hinges are installed temporarily in the locations previously marked. Further trimming may be necessary on the distal end of the thigh socket to allow free passage of the foot into the foot socket. Anteriorly the thigh socket is trimmed on its distal end to provide clearance for the heel tendon. If insufficient space is available to allow passage of the foot, a hinged panel is installed posteriorly on the distal end of the thigh socket.

To stabilize the anatomical knee within the thigh socket and to supply some degree of suspension, a 1½-in.-wide Velcro strap may be used. This strap is drawn through an aperture on the medial side of the thigh socket and passed around the stump just above the patella so as to pull the stump posteriorly. The strap continues through the lateral aperture, where it is fastened on the outside of the socket.

A modified Silesian belt of 1½-in. cotton webbing provides most of the suspension. A piece of San-splint* 2 in. wide and 4 in. long is molded over the opposite iliac crest, fitting around the anterior superior iliac spine for control of rotation.

Two areas of weight-bearing are provided in this prosthesis. One is at the ischial shelf, which is the primary source; the other is the long plantar ligament shelf (heel pad).

To ensure a stable knee without active extension of the anatomical foot on contact, the centers of knee hinges must be kept posterior to a plumb line between the trochanter and the ankle of the SACH foot.

Initially, the first prosthesis is fitted shorter than the sound leg and then lengthened according to the patient's progress during gait training.

Following completion of fitting and alignment procedures, final fabrication of the prosthesis is carried out with emphasis on cosmesis (Figures 18-A and 18-B). If a BK adjustable leg was used to obtain dynamic alignment (Figure 18-C), a transfer jig[†] is required in order to maintain alignment of the foot and upper section of the prosthesis. If alignment was done using filler blocks, these sections should be hollowed out to reduce the weight. In either case, the calf section is built up with Micro-Spheres[‡] or Hosmer Prosthetic Foam. The lower halves of the knee hinges are fastened permanently to the shank and a final lamination is applied to this part of the prosthesis. On the

*Available through Smith & Nephew, Lachine, Que.
†Hosmer Vertical Fabricating Jig, available through A. J. Hosmer Corp., Campbell, Calif.
‡Available through U.S. Manufacturing Co., Glendale, Calif.

thigh socket the upper halves of the knee hinges and the Silesian belt are removed. The holes left by the screws plus the side apertures are filled with wax. Final lamination of this section is carried out. Normally, no buildup of the top socket is required.

After lamination, the prosthesis is reassembled. The upper halves of the mechanical knee joints and the Silesian belt are riveted on after all the wax has been removed.

Figures 19-A through 19-E show stump and prosthesis before and after Van Nes osteotomy.

OTHER CONSIDERATIONS

Even when a good prosthesis has been supplied, the patient may still have a poor gait because of hip instability, and consideration should be given to reconstruction of the upper end of the femur in defects of Aitken's Types A and B. During the early years of life it may appear that no femoral head and neck are present; however, some hint can be obtained by determining whether or not the acetabulum seems to be developing normally. If there is a good acetabulum, then one can assume that a cartilaginous upper end of the femur is also present and will eventually ossify. When it does, a varus deformity of varying degrees of severity is seen.

Figures 20-A and 20-B and 21-A through 21-D demonstrate the type of deformity and the result obtained by osteotomy in two of our patients in the unilateral group. Two other patients also required an innominate osteotomy to render the hips stable because of an associated acetabular dysplasia.

In the patient with a very short distal femoral shaft only and no upper femoral end, consideration could be given to

fusion of this short shaft to the ischium or acetabulum with 180 deg of rotation of the lower fragment in order to use the knee joint as a hip and the ankle joint as a knee. This procedure has been performed in only one patient in the series of Toronto PFFD cases and that one has been done too recently for evaluation of the results.

SUMMARY

There are very many ways to approach the problem of the surgical and prosthetic management of a child with proximal femoral focal deficiency. The experience at the Amputee Clinic of the Ontario Crippled Children's Centre in Toronto has been outlined.

BIBLIOGRAPHY

1. Aitken, G. T. Instructional Course Lecture, American Academy of Orthopaedic Surgeons, 1967.
2. Amstutz, H. C., and P. D. Wilson. Dysgenesis of proximal femur (coxa vara) and the surgical management. J. Bone Joint Surg. 44A:1–24, 1962.
3. Bevan-Thomas, W. H., and E. A. Millar. A review of proximal focal femoral deficiencies. J. Bone Joint Surg. 49A(7):1376–1388, 1967.
4. Borggreve, J. Kniegelenksersatz durch das in der Beinlängsachse um 180° gedrehte Fussgelenk. Arch. Orthopäd. Chir. 28:175–178, 1930.
5. Van Nes, C. P. Rotation-plasty for congenital defects of the femur (making use of the ankle of the shortened limb to control the knee joint of a prosthesis. J. Bone Joint Surg. 32B:12–16, 1950.

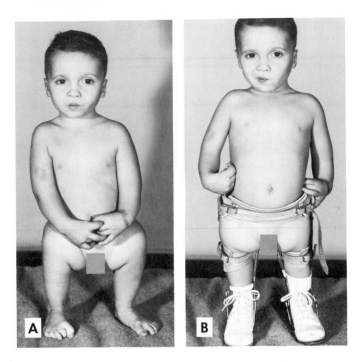

FIGURE 1-A   Three-year-old boy with bilateral proximal femoral focal deficiency and bilateral radial hemimelia.
FIGURE 1-B   Braces provided to keep hips and knees straight have increased his height by three inches. However, the braces were discarded because they severely handicapped him at play.

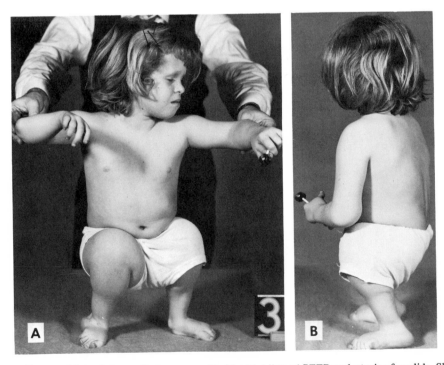

FIGURES 2-A and 2-B   Front and lateral views of a four-year-old girl with bilateral PFFD and ptosis of eyelids. She is also moderately retarded.

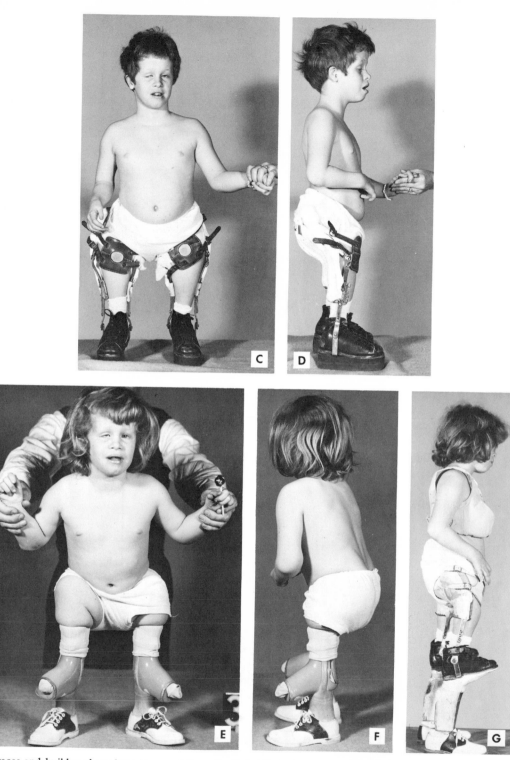

FIGURE 2-C   Braces and buildup shoes have increased the patient's height by four inches thus decreasing the leg-trunk disproportion, but also decreasing her function.

FIGURE 2-D   The plaster slab behind the thigh and buttocks holds the child erect without uncomfortable local pressure. Braces were rejected because of functional loss.

FIGURE 2-E   This simple type of extension prosthesis was the most satisfactory type of appliance from the patient's viewpoint.

FIGURE 2-F   Lateral view of the extension prostheses showing the girl's flexed hips and the back of knee joints in the apparatus.

FIGURE 2-G   This more complicated prosthesis in which plantar flexion of the ankle substituted for knee flexion was not completely successful, and is now being modified by having the feet in less fixed dorsiflexion.

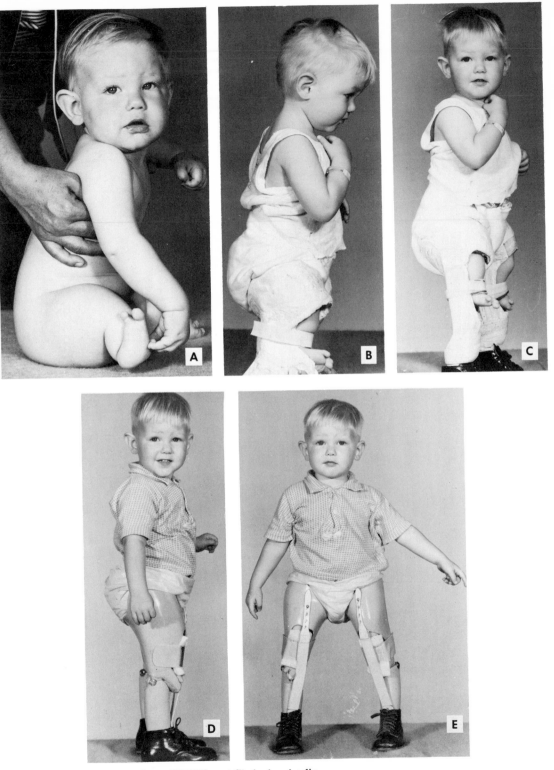

FIGURE 3-A   Two-year-old boy with bilateral PFFD's and fibular hemimelia.

FIGURE 3-B   The boy's first prosthesis; a simple set of plaster "stubbies."

FIGURE 3-C   The plaster prostheses have been lengthened and he enjoys being at the same height as his friends. He is very agile and his function is good.

FIGURE 3-D   Knee joints have been added to normalize sitting. The posterior hinge placement makes knee very stable and the boy wears the limbs for most of the day.

FIGURE 3-E   Anterior view showing wide base gait. Extension straps increase knee stability.

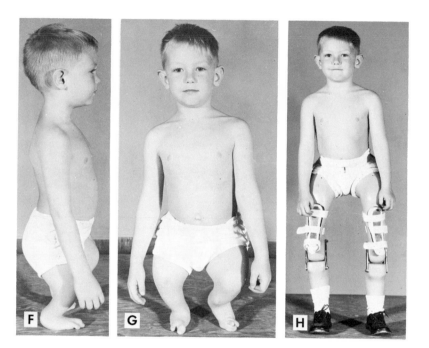

FIGURE 3-F   Function out of prostheses is so good that it precludes any thought of active knee control by rotation osteotomy.
FIGURE 3-G   Although feet are small and deformed, this boy is extremely agile and uses all four limbs when he runs.
FIGURE 3-H   At age seven he has learned an effective bilateral knee-disarticulation gait which has been aided by the recent addition of
OCCC stable knee joints.

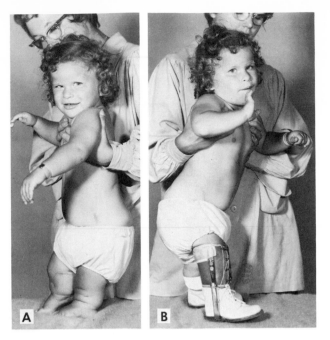

FIGURE 4-A   This retarded child has bilateral PFFD associated with severe clubfeet (partially corrected) and hypoplastic tibiae.
FIGURE 4-B   Walking was not possible for this child with a pair of simple braces.

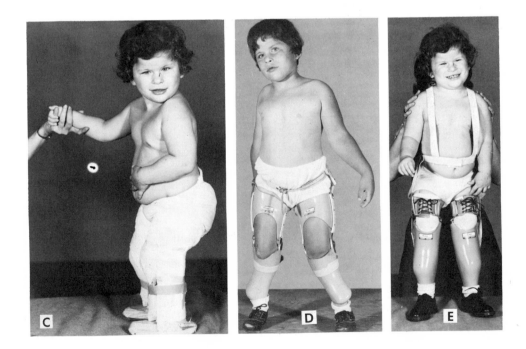

FIGURE 4-C   A molded pair of plaster stubbies gives enough stability to stand and begin walking.
FIGURE 4-D   The presence of deformed feet made prosthetic fitting difficult. Ambulation without her prostheses was not possible.
FIGURE 4-E   After Syme's amputations, function and appearance in prostheses are improved, and function out of prostheses is
unaltered.

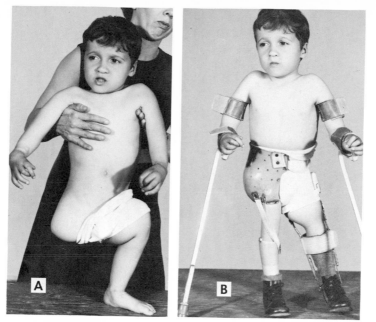

FIGURE 5-A   Five-year-old boy with left PFFD, right amelia, and bilateral radial hemimelia.
FIGURE 5-B   Independent ambulation has been attained with hip-disarticulation prosthesis, extension brace, and special crutches.

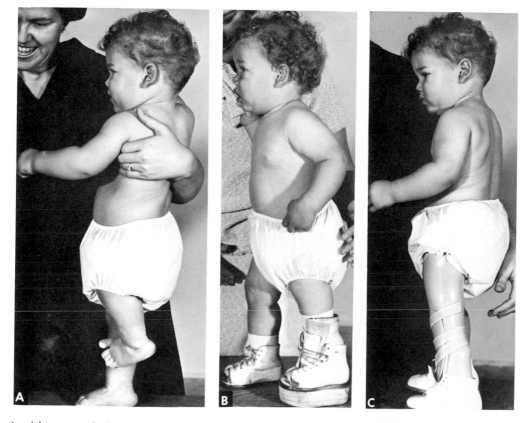

FIGURE 6-A   An eighteen-month-old boy with a typical unilateral PFFD and no associated defects.
FIGURE 6-B   The first prosthesis was an O'Connor boot with sole raises added as he grew.
FIGURE 6-C   A plastic-laminated extension prosthesis with the foot held in nearly full plantar flexion. Anterior aperture provides access.

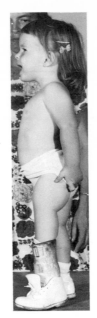

FIGURE 7   An O'Connor boot provided for a 3½" leg-length discrepancy. Velcro straps replace usual anterior lacing.

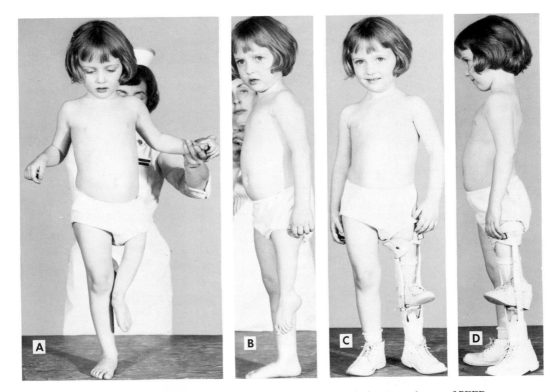

FIGURE 8-A   This girl shows the wide perineum and very short femur indicative of a severe degree of PFFD.
FIGURE 8-B   Her ankle is very mobile with a range of almost 90 deg.
FIGURE 8-C   The type of brace worn when first seen at our clinic.
FIGURE 8-D   Function was good for active control of knee flexion and extension using ankle, but girl was very unhappy about the
    appearance of her leg.

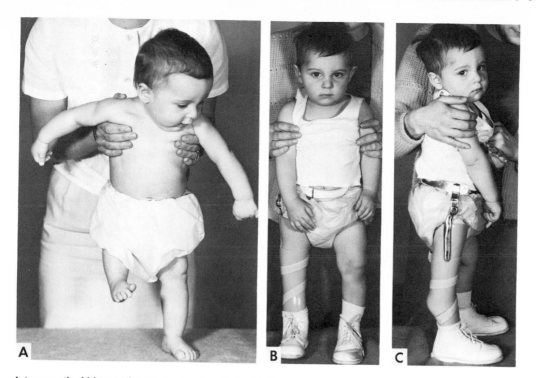

FIGURE 9-A   A ten-month-old boy trying to stand and ready for his first prosthesis.
FIGURE 9-B   The same boy at 18 months of age gets along very well on his extension prosthesis and finds it a problem only when sitting, kneeling, or trying to ride a bicycle.
FIGURE 9-C   A lateral view of limb showing pelvic band used to control a tendency toward external rotation. The anterior window cover is held in by a spiral Velcro strap.

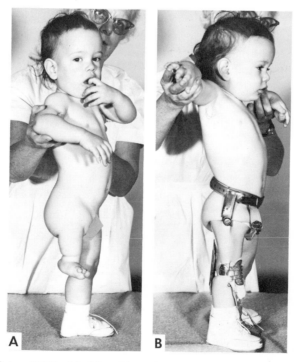

FIGURE 10-A   PFFD with right ankle nearly at level of left knee.
FIGURE 10-B   A passive knee joint has been supplied in the form of outside hinges.

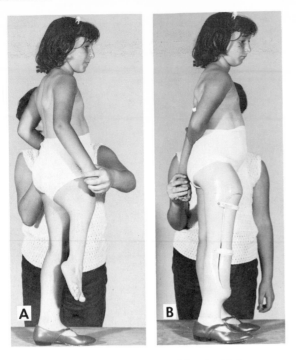

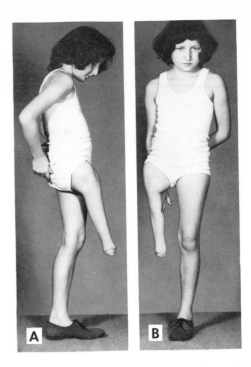

FIGURE 11-A   An older girl whose parents did not wish to
consider surgical conversion.
FIGURE 11-B   Even with hip- and knee-flexion deformities and
incomplete plantar flexion, an extension prosthesis with reasonably smooth contours can be made.

FIGURE 12-A   Syme's amputation and repair of varus deformity
of neck of femur have given this girl a stump which can be fitted
with a knee-disarticulation-type prosthesis.
FIGURE 12-B   In this girl the PFFD was associated with a paraxial
fibular hemimelia with a poor ankle joint and foot, and a deformity of the right hand (syndactyly).

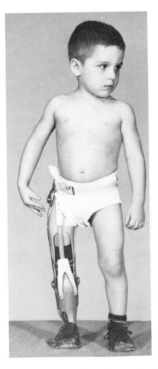

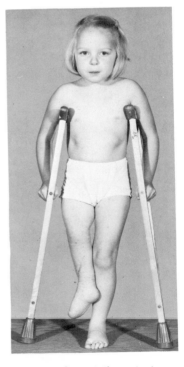

FIGURE 13   This lad had a tibial rotation osteotomy at the age of
three years. A pelvic band and a hip joint were added to help
prevent derotation, but a repeat osteotomy was necessary after
2½ years.

FIGURE 14   Two years after rotation osteotomy of tibia, this girl
had lost 60 deg of rotation. Level of knee joint was improved at
second osteotomy by resection of three inches of tibia.

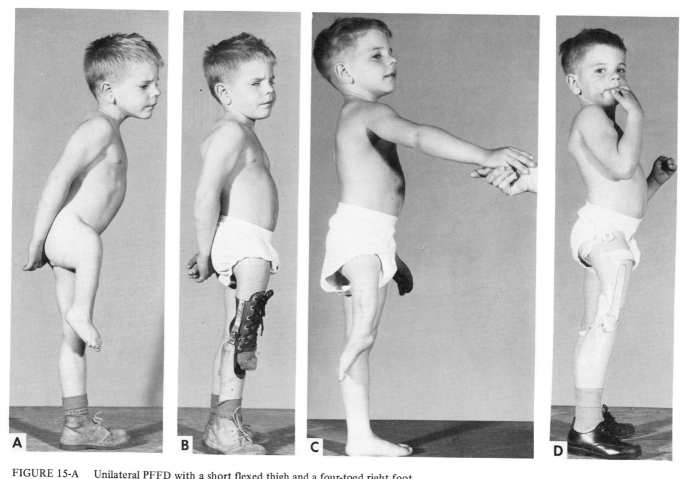

FIGURE 15-A Unilateral PFFD with a short flexed thigh and a four-toed right foot.
FIGURE 15-B Original prosthesis with a passive knee joint below the heel.
FIGURE 15-C The appearance of the leg after a one-stage tibial rotation osteotomy.
FIGURE 15-D Prosthesis fitted after rotation osteotomy has good cosmetic appearance and active knee control from full extension to 75 deg of flexion. Most satisfactory gain for this boy was ability to ride an ordinary bicycle with standard pedals.

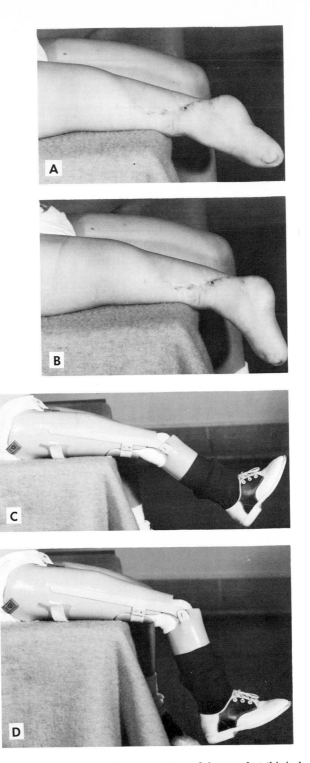

FIGURE 16-A   The appearance of the stump can be improved by amputation of the toes, but this is done at the expense of some loss in power and increased initial morbidity.

FIGURE 16-B   Showing the range of active ankle dorsiflexion or, as the child soon learns to think of it, "knee flexion."

FIGURE 16-C   A slight extension lag is apparent when the prosthesis is extended against gravity, but not while standing on leg. Detail of the prosthesis is shown. The most difficult part of fitting is in the placement of the knee joint.

FIGURE 16-D   Active knee flexion is shown one week after fitting of prosthesis. When child kneels, further passive flexion is possible by stump sliding partially out of socket.

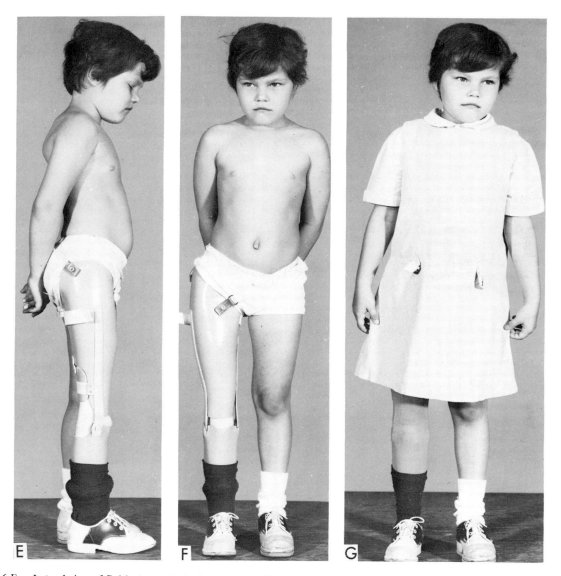

FIGURE 16-E   Lateral view of finished prosthesis. Strap at rear of thigh is inside suspension strap which fits just over patella. Window at
rear aids in access and suspension.

FIGURE 16-F   The slight difference in knee level has not been a functional problem and can be managed later, if necessary, at time of knee
arthrodesis. Pelvic strap which aids in rotation control and suspension is often not necessary.

FIGURE 16-G   Cosmetic appearance is satisfactory in clothing.

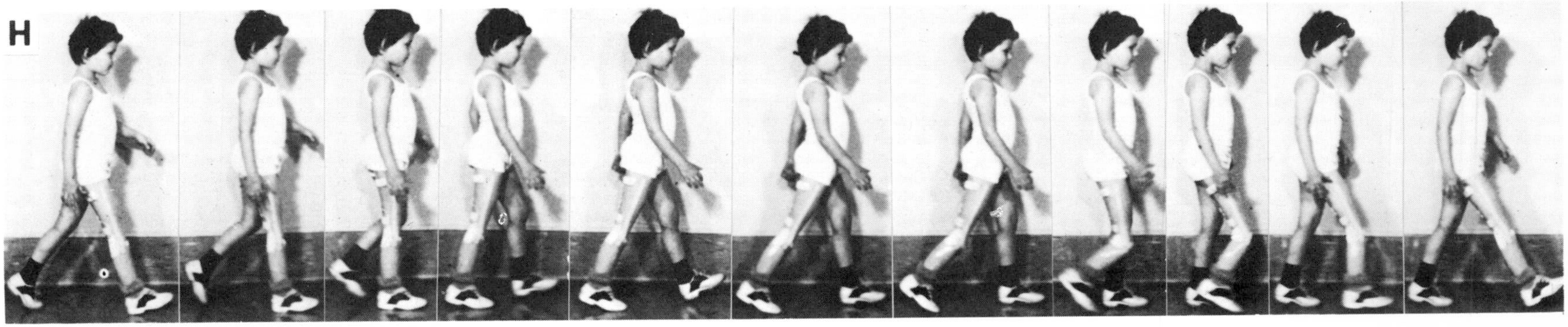

FIGURE 16-H   Frames from movie of child shown in Figures 16-A through 16-G.

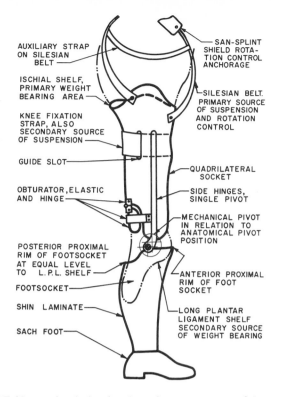

AUXILIARY STRAP ON SILESIAN BELT

ISCHIAL SHELF, PRIMARY WEIGHT BEARING AREA

KNEE FIXATION STRAP, ALSO SECONDARY SOURCE OF SUSPENSION

GUIDE SLOT

OBTURATOR, ELASTIC AND HINGE

POSTERIOR PROXIMAL RIM OF FOOTSOCKET AT EQUAL LEVEL TO L.P.L. SHELF

FOOTSOCKET

SHIN LAMINATE

SACH FOOT

SAN-SPLINT SHIELD ROTA-TION CONTROL ANCHORAGE

SILESIAN BELT. PRIMARY SOURCE OF SUSPENSION AND ROTATION CONTROL

QUADRILATERAL SOCKET

SIDE HINGES, SINGLE PIVOT

MECHANICAL PIVOT IN RELATION TO ANATOMICAL PIVOT POSITION

ANTERIOR PROXIMAL RIM OF FOOT SOCKET

LONG PLANTAR LIGAMENT SHELF SECONDARY SOURCE OF WEIGHT BEARING

FIGURE 17   A sketch showing the various components of the prosthesis.

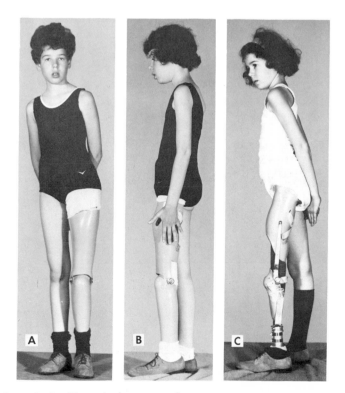

FIGURE 18-A   Completed prosthesis with emphasis on cosmesis.
FIGURE 18-B   Lateral view of same prosthesis shows no panel behind knee as adequate suspension was provided by knee strap.
FIGURE 18-C   The jig stage of fitting is essential to ensure proper knee-joint placement and alignment.

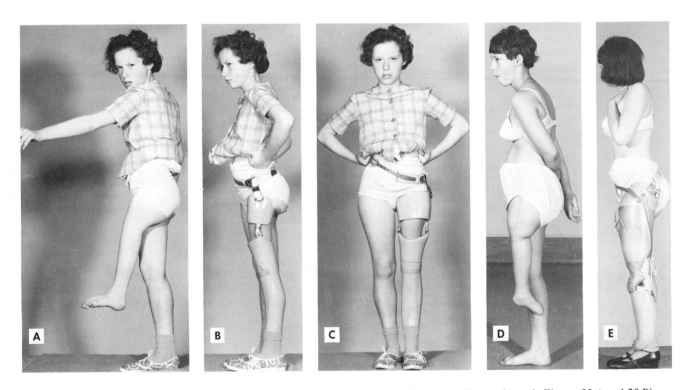

FIGURE 19-A   Unilateral PFFD in a 12-year-old girl who has had surgical repair of coxa vara (x-rays shown in Figures 20-A and 20-B).

FIGURE 19-B   Original prosthesis with joints at level of anatomical hip and knee. Function was good, but she was concerned about appearance, particularly when sitting.

FIGURE 19-C   Anterior view of original prosthesis.

FIGURE 19-D   Rotation of limb has been done through knee arthrodesis; toes were removed at same time.

FIGURE 19-E   Appearance of final prosthesis is satisfactory and knee is at correct level. She took many months to obtain as good function as she had before rotation arthrodesis.

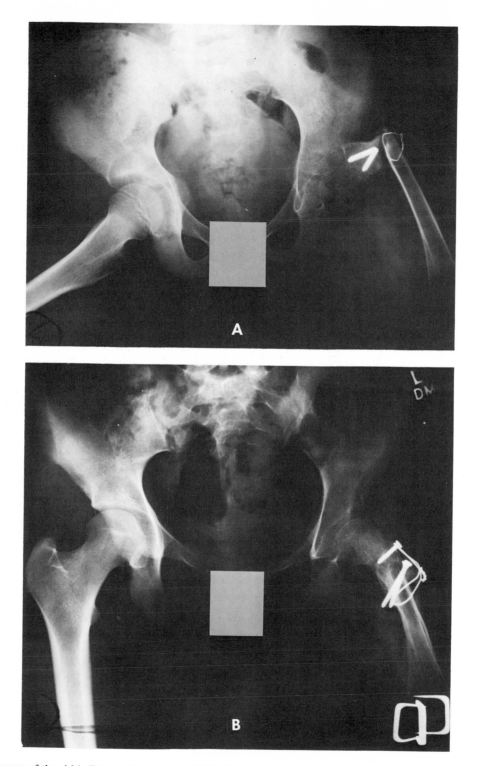

FIGURE 20-A   An x-ray of the girl in Figures 19-A through 19-E. Three previous attempts at repair of the hip had failed. There was a cartilaginous defect at the intertrochanteric level with pain in the hip after strenuous activity.

FIGURE 20-B   Three years after repair the shape of the femoral neck is good although the acetabulum is somewhat dysplastic. Two other children who have had similar femoral repairs have had innominate osteotomies, but are too early postoperative to assess.

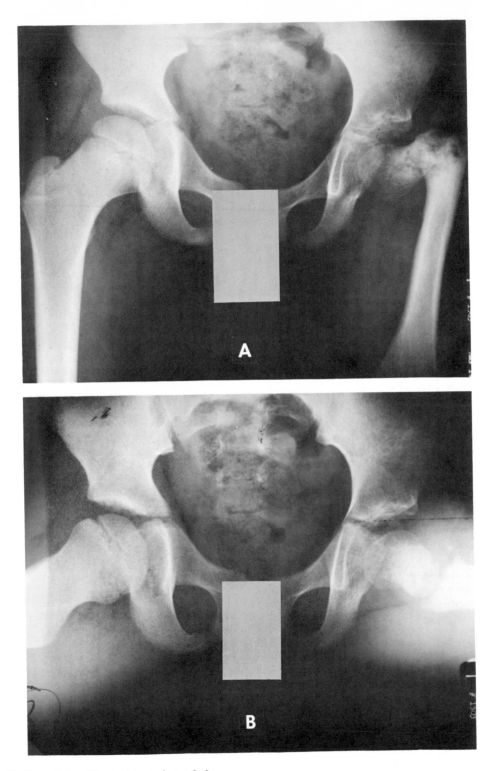

FIGURE 21-A   PFFD with good acetabulum.
FIGURE 21-B   PFFD with cartilaginous defect at base of femoral neck below greater trochanter.

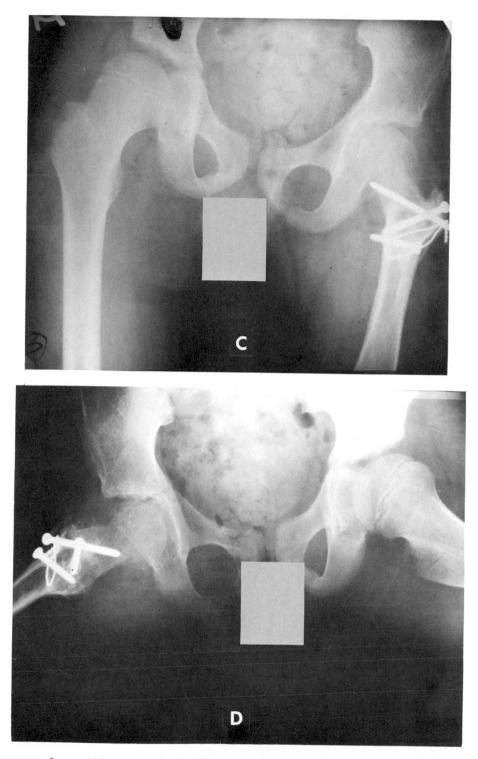

FIGURE 21-C   Four years after surgical reconstruction the hip is stable with good muscle control, a full range of movement, and a negative Trendelenburg.

FIGURE 21-D   Postoperative view shows slight retroversion but good remodeling and a congruous joint.

G. WILBUR WESTIN, M.D.
FINN O. GUNDERSON, M.D.

PROXIMAL FEMORAL FOCAL DEFICIENCY–
A Review of Treatment Experiences

To evaluate the treatment of proximal femoral focal deficiency (PFFD), 165 cases of this relatively uncommon anomaly have been reviewed. It was believed that by gathering cases from all of the Shriners Hospitals, reviewing the history and treatment of these patients, and reporting on composite experience, a rational approach to this difficult problem would evolve. In the past, treatment had involved the accommodation of the deformity in some type of prosthesis or brace. Collective experience now favors early elimination of the defect by surgical conversion to an amputation-type stump which provides improved function and cosmesis.

MATERIAL

All seventeen units of the Shriners Hospitals for Crippled Children contributed detailed information on 165 cases of PFFD. These cases were located with the help of the central office in Chicago, where computer records of all Shriners Hospital patients, past and present, are located. A total of 400 patient records were reviewed by the doctors in each unit, and those falling into the category of PFFD were reported in detail. Further information, including copies of operative reports, x-rays, and progress notes, was obtained. Treatment has ranged from prosthetic fitting alone to multiple surgical procedures. Of the 165 patients in the PFFD category, 70 were treated without surgery and 95 with surgery. The surgical approach to these 95 patients was evaluated in detail.

THE DISEASE STATE

The etiology of PFFD is unknown. It is known that the development of the limb buds takes place early in fetal life, beginning at about four weeks' gestation. Various factors act upon the developing limb, resulting in rotation, segmentation, longitudinal growth, and differentiation of elements. The most proximal elements of the limb develop first (4, 6), and the hand and foot follow, being fully formed by the seventh week. Chemical toxicity (6), radiation (6), enzyme alterations, viral infections (6), and mechanical trauma (10) have produced limb anomalies in humans and experimental animals. Ring (14, 15) has stated that the primary problem is in the enchondral ossification of defective cartilage. Gardner (6) pointed out that failure of skeletal elements to form may be due to factors operating during the period of differentiation. This critical period—at four to eight weeks of fetal life—was defined by studies of thalidomide babies. It is apparent from these and other studies that as the severity of the defect increases, so does the incidence of associated anomalies. A multifocal process must be supposed, and it must act over a period of time, the severity and variety of involvement increasing with the duration of the process. The frequency (50 percent) of congenital absence of the fibula in cases of PFFD (Table 1) supports this theory, since the more distal portions of the limb develop last.

The theory advanced by Morgan and Somerville (10), that mechanical trauma to the advancing growth plate interferes with the development of normal infantile valgus, may be appropriate for simple coxa vara, but it does not explain

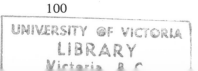

TABLE 1   Associated Anomalies (in percentage)

Total incidence of other defects	65
Congenital absence of the fibula, same leg	50
Contralateral leg anomalies	26
Arm anomalies	26
Other congenital defects	9

the wide dissociation of fragments seen in the typical case of PFFD. Among the unexplained features of this anomaly is the frequent presence in the acetabulum of a vestigial femoral head, often completely dissociated from a small shaft element. Perhaps the head has a separate impetus to develop associated with its position in the acetabulum. Review of the prenatal and familial history in these patients reveals no consistent factor. Breech presentation was the only frequently recorded variation from normal (18 percent). Two cases of nonidentical twins were found, and in each set only one of the twins had phocomelia. There is one reference to a set of twins (*14*) with phocomelia present in both children. This variability raises the question of individual susceptibility, whatever the cause. We believe that the evidence points to an etiology extrinsic to the fetus.

THE CLINICAL PICTURE

The deformity is commonly noted at birth. The thigh is shortened and bulky. There are usually flexion contractures of the hip and knee. After the patient learns to walk, there is a short-leg gait, a gluteus medius limp, and the foot is in equinus. Relative shortening of the extremity is progressive, carrying the knee higher and higher. In mild cases, early x-rays may show absence of the capital femoral epiphysis and a normal femoral shaft. This picture often leads to an erroneous diagnosis of congenital dislocation of the hip (Figure 1-A).

The deformity makes bracing or prosthetic fitting increasingly difficult. The hip- and knee-flexion contractures and associated anomalies contribute to the orthotic problem. Symptoms are related to the shortening of the limb and hip instability. Hip pain is seldom a complaint (*9*). In spite of the complete separation of the shaft from proximal elements, little or no telescoping occurs with weight-bearing. Apparently the short rotators and iliopsoas contribute to this stability. The abductor lurch is quite prominent.

TREATMENT

Since 1950 the majority of these patients have been treated surgically. The purpose of the surgery has been to: (1) improve prosthetic fitting and use, (2) improve hip stability

and prevent increasing deformity, and (3) equalize leg lengths.

Amputation, knee arthrodesis, and occasionally rotation osteotomy have been used to help prosthetic fit and use. Leg lengthening has been attempted with little real success. Hip surgery has included a number of procedures, the most common being valgus osteotomy. Arthroplasty has not been a success in reconstituting a satisfactory femoral-acetabular joint. Soft tissue release at the knee or hip done solely for flexion contracture has failed repeatedly!

AMPUTATION

The most common procedure has been amputation, which was performed on 59 patients (Table 2). The Syme's type of ankle disarticulation has been the most satisfactory operation performed. Four of the below-knee and one of the foot amputations (a Chopart's) required revision. The goal of amputation is a long, above-knee, end-bearing stump that can be easily fitted in a standard prosthesis.

TABLE 2   Amputation Levels

Syme's amputation	32	Revisions	0
Below-knee amputation	16	Revisions	4
Foot amputation distal to ankle joint	9	Revisions	1
Bilateral Syme's amputation	2	Revisions	0
Total amputations	59		

KNEE ARTHRODESIS

Knee arthrodesis was performed on 31 patients (Table 3). Amputation accompanied the arthrodesis in 25 of these cases. It was found that after knee arthrodesis in full extension, the hip-flexion contracture was spontaneously corrected. One or both of the epiphyses at the knee can be excised, the goal being a long above-knee stump at maturity. Two knee fusions were considered delayed unions after the patients fell during the healing process, requiring further immobilization to achieve union.

TABLE 3   Knee Arthrodesis

With Syme's amputation	16
Without amputation	5
With below-knee amputation	7
Bilateral with bilateral Syme's	2
Bilateral without amputation	1
Total arthrodesis	31
Delayed union	2

LEG LENGTHENING

Leg lengthening has been attempted in nine cases with little success and frequent complications (Table 4). In no instance was leg length equalized. One of the criteria (18) for consideration of femoral lengthening is the presence of a stable hip and knee rarely found in PFFD.

TABLE 4   Leg-Lengthening Procedures

Total patients	9
Total operations	14
Femoral lengthening operations	13
Tibial lengthening operations	1
Operations gained 1 in. or more	6
Patients with complications	8
Leg length equalized	0

ROTATION OSTEOTOMY

Eight patients have had the Borggreve rotational osteotomy (as described by Van Nes, 17) or a modification thereof (Table 5). This operation externally rotates the foot 180 deg by tibial or femoral osteotomy so that the ankle joint functions as a knee joint. Power from the plantar flexors is used to extend the prosthetic leg. Attaining 180 deg of rotation usually requires two or more operations and frequently many months in the hospital. In our group of cases, only two of the eight patients so treated can be classified as successful. Two cases were complete failures, necessitating return to the original position. The other four patients failed to gain full rotation. The cosmetic deformity of a foot

TABLE 5   Rotational Osteotomy

Total patients	8
Total operations	16
180° rotation achieved	2 patients
Failure	2 patients
Less than full rotation	4 patients

pointing the wrong way could be distressing to some patients, especially girls. This, together with the prolonged treatment time, may outweigh the functional advantage.

EXCISION OF THE FEMORAL FRAGMENT

In nine patients the proximal end of the tibia was placed into the acetabulum after excision of the short femoral fragment (Table 6). Deepening of the acetabulum accompanied four of these transfers. The growing tibial epiphysis tends to accommodate to the shape of the acetabulum. The procedure is usually accompanied by Syme's amputation. The abductors, when present, are transferred distally on the shaft of the tibia to give added abductor strength.

The patients had a decreased range of motion and especially had decreased flexion power in the reconstructed hip joint. In the more severe types of PFFD there may be no acetabulum. Without an acetabulum, we would caution against this type of conversion.

PROXIMAL FEMORAL OSTEOTOMY

The most common surgical procedure at the hip joint was subtrochanteric valgus osteotomy (Table 7). These proce-

TABLE 6   Excision of the Femoral Fragment[a]

Unit No.	Patient No.	Age	Date	Procedure	Result
1	5224	4 yr	1954	Simple excision of femur	Instability persisted. "Rating excellent, with good gait."
1	6204	3 yr	1965	Simple excision of femur.	Excessive motion at hip. Rated satisfactory.
1	6759	5 yr	1959	Simple excision of femur.	"Gait good, rating good."
12	4404	6 yr	1958	Femur excised, Colonna arthroplasty over tibia.	Hip stable with good extension power.
12	4659	5 yr	1957	Simple excision of femur.	Good stability with strong extension power.
12	8798	4 yr	1960	Simple excision of femur.	Operative tachycardia. Died night of surgery.
12	9223	2 yr	1960	Simple excision of femur.	Increased stability. Proximal tibia well seated on x-ray.
12	9485	5 yr	1961	Excision of femur. Proximal tibia shaped and placed into acetabulum.	Both hips stable. Flexion weak on left. Transfer of rectus abdominis in 1966 to increase flexion power of left hip partially successful.
		6 yr	1962	Bilateral procedures.	
12	9936	1 yr	1963	Excision of femur and tibial-acetabular arthroplasty.	Hip stable with negative Trendelenberg. Flexion limited to 15 deg.

[a]When excision of the femoral fragment is accompanied by arthroplasty, stability is increased. Good extension power is retained, but flexion is weak. Excision of the femoral fragment eliminates the hip- and knee-flexion contractures.

TABLE 7   Proximal Femoral Osteotomy

Unit No.	Patient No.	Age	Date	Procedure	Result
1	1175	9 yr	1931	"Osteotomy for varus."	Unknown.
1	6205	4 yr	1957	Subtrochanteric closing wedge valgus osteotomy.	Failed.
		7 yr	1960	Repeat same operation.	Successful with six-year follow-up.
1	6991	7 yr	1962	Valgus osteotomy of proximal femoral shaft.	Unknown.
1	7634	13 yr	1958	Anterior angulation osteotomy.	Done to realign the hip fused in flexion.
4	2706	9 yr	1958	Subtrochanteric valgus osteotomy.	Failed.
		12 yr	1961	Valgus subtrochanteric osteotomy with blade plate.	Plate broke, failed varus of 75 deg.
6	12	8 yr	1954	Intertrochanteric closing wedge osteotomy.	Corrected 80 to 130 deg. Hip later degenerated.
6		4 yr	1957	Subtrochanteric valgus osteotomy.	Failed.
		6 yr	1959	Repeat with 165 deg blade plate.	Corrected to 150 deg with 7-year follow-up.
6	988	3 yr	1960	Inverted-V valgus osteotomy.	Failed.
		4 yr	1961	Valgus subtrochanteric osteotomy fixed with Steinmann pins.	Failed.
		8 yr	1964	Excision of neck defect with shaft fixed to head.	Position of 135 deg maintained 2 yr.
6	1432	3 yr	1963	Subtrochanteric valgus osteotomy.	Failed.
		5 yr	1965	Repeat.	105 to 125 deg maintained 1 yr to date.
6	1971	8 yr	1965	Subtrochanteric valgus osteotomy.	85 to 165 deg maintained for 1 yr.
9	7410	14 yr	1957	Subtrochanteric valgus osteotomy.	Failed.
9	8550	3 yr	1962	Lateral closing wedge valgus subtrochanteric osteotomy.	85 to 115 deg later failed.
		7 yr	1966	Valgus osteotomy with Blount blade plate fix.	Successful to date.
12	3605	8 yr	1949	Subtrochanteric valgus osteotomy.	Nonunion, grafted, failed.
13	2189	5 yr	1963	Varus osteotomy to seat the shaft better.	Increased stability.
15	8170	5 yr	1964	Lateral closing wedge valgus subtrochanteric osteotomy.	80 to 110 deg maintained for 2 yr.
15	5370	7 yr	1947	Subtrochanteric osteotomy.	Done to realign the leg after fusion, success.
15	9178	6 yr	1964	Subtrochanteric valgus osteotomy.	Failed.
		6 yr	1964	Repeat.	Minimal or no correction.
16	6361	7 yr	1962	Subtrochanteric lateral closing wedge osteotomy.	60 to 90 deg improvement.

Summary of Results

Total patients	18
Total osteotomies	26
Success	9
Failure	11
Result unknown	7

dures have been successful in correcting varus in only one-third of the operations performed. The low success rate is attributed to failure to recognize the abnormal anatomy of the femur at the time of osteotomy. Some hips have no femoral head ossification or significant development of the acetabulum. Others have an intact cartilaginous continuity from the short femoral shaft to the ossifying femoral head. In all our cases where such a cartilaginous bridge was present, osteotomy was unsuccessful (Figures 1-A through 1-G). Only when ossification of the femoral head, neck, and shaft have progressed to bony continuity at the site of osteotomy (Figures 2-A, 2-B, and 2-C), or when the cartilaginous portion can be excised to produce bony continuity, will this procedure be successful.

The success rate of the osteotomies done to correct varus was directly related to the amount of unossified cartilage between the head and the shaft, and to the age of the patients. A fair success rate was achieved in coxa vara with

shortening where the growth plate was narrow. In those cases where a wide, abnormal cartilaginous bridge was present, the osteotomy always failed—the pin or plate pulled out of the cartilage and the fixation was lost. Further ossification occurs with age, and the defect can then be excised with fusion of the neck or head of the femur to the shaft in valgus. This procedure is usually possible by the age of eight to ten years. The abnormal proximal growth plate does not represent a significant consideration.

ARTHROPLASTY OF THE HIP

In nine patients, attempts were made to obtain increased stability of the hip by arthroplasty. Six of the thirteen operations performed were reported as increasing stability (Table 8). Four of these were in the previously mentioned cases where excision of the femoral fragment was followed

TABLE 8   Arthroplasty of the Hip

Unit No.	Patient No.	Age	Date	Procedure	Result
6	179	10 yr	1953	Fascia lata shaft arthroplasty.	Operated hip stiffer than other in this bilateral case. Poor result.
6	1115	9 yr	1963	Fascia lata shaft arthroplasty with Pemberton osteotomy.	Hip dislocated. Result poor.
		10 yr	1963	Adult-type Colonna arthroplasty.	Redislocated, open reduction and fixation. Hip stiff.
9	3344	12 yr	1949	Greater trochanter into acetabulum, left hip (bilateral case).	Result unknown.
		13 yr	1950	Mold arthroplasty right hip shaft.	Flexion 30/40, abduction 15/20, IR 0/0, ExR 60/50.
		13 yr	1950	Mold shaft arthroplasty left hip.	Marked waddle bilateral at age 16.
12	3370	12 yr	1957	Femur absent. Proximal tibia placed in acetabulum.	Result satisfactory. "Walks well for short distances."
12	4404	8 yr	1960	Colonna arthroplasty.	Good initial stability with good extension power.
12		18 mo	1958	Greater trochanter placed in acetabulum.	Failed.
		4 yr	1961	Colonna arthroplasty.	Foot externally rotated. Hip stiff and painful.
12	9485	5 yr	1961	Tibial–acetabular arthroplasty, right (bilateral case).	Hip stable with good power. Good result.
		6 yr	1962	Tibial–acetabular arthroplasty, left.	Hip stable. Weak flexion. Rectus abdominis transfer 1966 to strengthen flexion.
12	9936	1 yr	1963	Tibial–acetabular arthroplasty.	Good stability. Negative Trendelenberg test. Flexion 0 to 15 deg.
14	105	3 yr	1927	Trochanter into acetabulum.	Operative death, no autopsy.

by acetabular deepening. One patient died during surgery. Bilateral procedures were performed in two cases. In one of these, mold-shaft arthroplasty apparently gave a fair result. Two fascia lata arthroplasties were failures. In the remaining cases the acetabulum was cleared of bone remnants and fibrous tissue and the proximal femoral shaft or trochanter reduced into it. Only one of these was reported as having a good result.

Evaluation of these results is difficult; hence, status has been indicated as accurately as possible, or questionnaire has been quoted. It appears that the majority of these procedures have not been successful in increasing function. In only one was the Trendelenberg test negative.

HIP ARTHRODESIS

Hip arthrodesis has not usually been a beneficial procedure (Table 9). Such a procedure is contraindicated if a prosthesis is to be fitted on the same side.

TABLE 9   Arthrodesis of the Hip

Unit No.	Patient No.	Age	Date	Procedure	Result
3	3608	9½ yr	1949	Arthrodesis, right hip.	Fusion failed. Motion was painless with moderate pistoning at age 20.
12	2448	11 yr	1949	"Bosworth" arthrodesis, left hip.	Failed. Peroneal nerve palsy a complication.
4	1748	4 yr	1954	Bilateral arthrodesis with hips externally rotated.	180-deg rotation was the goal to use the knee as a hip joint. This failed and hips were rotated back. Final result was a patient with buttocks 1 ft off ground.
15	5370	9 yr	1947	Arthrodesis, left hip.	Fused in too much flexion. Osteotomy done to correct this but left at 50 deg. Patient had below-knee amputation. He walks but has back strain.
8	3020	10 yr	1961	Arthrodesis, left hip.	Three subsequent rotation osteotomies. Patient can only walk with crutches, with marked lurching. Poor result.

CONCLUSIONS AND RECOMMENDATIONS

Most of the Shriners Hospitals' surgeons have struggled through similar patterns of treatment. The following recommendations are made as a result of this review:

Hip Joint: No surgery except subtrochanteric osteotomy in the presence of (or being able to obtain) bone continuity of the femoral neck and shaft.
Excision of the femoral fragment has produced a satisfactory result in a few cases, especially when accompanied by acetabuloplasty. It should be considered only in the more severe cases where there is no proximal continuity, as it precludes the possibility of performing other procedures for hip stability should future bone development unite the femoral head to the shaft.

Knee Joint: Arthrodesis in full extension. Excise (neither, one, or both) adjacent epiphyses dependent upon projected future growth.
Knee fusion provides a stable extremity in good alignment under the pelvis and well suited for fitting an above-knee prosthesis. Enough bone should be removed to obtain full extension at the operating table without soft tissue release. Postoperatively it may be necessary to cast the involved extremity in considerable flexion and/or abduction. However, after removal of the cast, the extremity readily assumes full extension, thereby correcting flexion contractures of the hip as well as the knee joint.

Ankle: Disarticulation using the heel pad for end-bearing.
The Syme's-type ankle disarticulation provides excellent end-bearing and simplifies the fitting of a prosthesis.

Prosthesis: The prosthesis should be designed for end-bearing (total-contact socket).
Conversion of the patient to an amputee is recommended as soon as the growth potential of the extremity can be determined with reasonable accuracy. This should be done before the child attends school and hopefully may make it possible for him to proceed in an unrestricted fashion throughout growth and development.

ACKNOWLEDGMENT

The authors wish to express appreciation to each unit of the Shriners Hospitals for contributions of information and participation in the analysis of the data contained in this paper.

BIBLIOGRAPHY

1. Aitken, G. T. Amputation as a treatment for certain lower-extremity congenital abnormalities. J. Bone Joint Surg. 41A(7): 1267–1285, 1959.
2. Amstutz, H. C., and P. D. Wilson, Jr. Dysgenesis of the proximal femur (coxa vara) and its surgical management. J. Bone Joint Surg. 44A(1):1–24, 1962.
3. Babb, F. S., R. K. Ghormley, and C. C. Chatterton. Congenital coxa vara. J. Bone Joint Surg. 31A:115–131, 1949.
4. Borggreve, J., Kniegelenksersatz durch das in der Beinlängsachse um 180° gedrehte Fussgelenk. Arch. Orthopäd. Chir. 28:175–178, 1930.
5. Frantz, C. H., and R. O'Rahilly. Congenital skeletal limb deficiencies. J. Bone Joint Surg. 43A(8):1202–1224, 1961.
6. Gardner, E. D. The development and growth of bones and joints. A.A.O.S. Instructional Course Lecture. J. Bone Joint Surg. 45A(4):856–862, 1963.
7. Golding, F. C. Congenital coxa vara. J. Bone Joint Surg. 30B(1): 161–163, 1948.
8. Lloyd-Roberts, G. C., and K. H. Stone. Congenital hypoplasia of the upper femur. J. Bone Joint Surg. 45B(3):557–560, 1963.
9. Mital, M. A., K. S. Masalawalla, and M. G. Desai. Bilateral congenital aplasia of the femur. J. Bone Joint Surg. 45B(3):561–565, 1963.
10. Morgan, J. D., and E. W. Somerville. Normal and abnormal growth at the upper end of the femur. J. Bone Joint Surg. 42B:264–272, 1960.
11. Noble, T. P., and E. D. Hauser. Coxa vara. Arch. Surg. 12:501–538, 1926.
12. Ollerenshaw, R. Congenital defects of the long bones of the lower limb. J. Bone Joint Surg. 7:528–552, 1925.
13. O'Rahilly, R. The development and the developmental disturbances of the limbs. Irish J. Med. Sci., No. 397:30–33, 1959.
14. Ring, P. A. Congenital short femur. J. Bone Joint Surg. 41B: 73–79, 1959.
15. Ring, P. A. Congenital abnormalities of the femur. Arch. Dis. Child. 36:410–417, 1961.
16. Trueta, J. The normal vascular anatomy of the human femoral head during growth. J. Bone Joint Surg. 39B:358–394, 1957.
17. Van Nes, C. P. Rotation-plasty for congenital defects of femur. J. Bone Joint Surg. 32B:12–16, 1950.
18. Westin, G. W. Femoral lengthening using a periosteal sleeve. J. Bone Joint Surg. 49A(5):836–854, 1967.
19. Wood, W. L., N. Zlotsky, and G. W. Westin. Congenital absence of the fibula; treatment by Syme amputation—indications and technique. J. Bone Joint Surg. 47A(6):1159–1169, 1965.

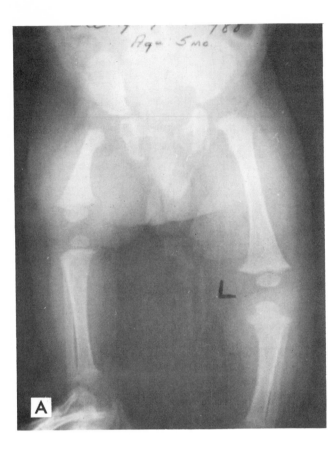

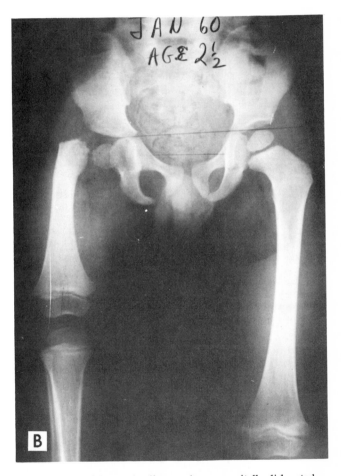

FIGURE 1-A   Proximal femoral focal deficiency prior to ossification of either femoral head; may be diagnosed as congenitally dislocated
hip.
FIGURE 1-B   Same case at age two years, seven months; note cartilaginous defect in trochanteric area.

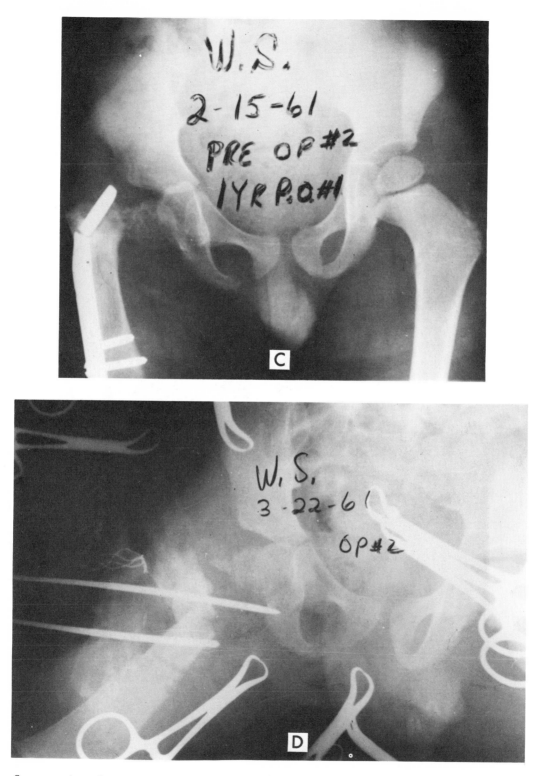

FIGURE 1-C   Same case at age three years, eight months; one year after trochanteric osteotomy—unsuccessful.
FIGURE 1-D   Same case at age three years, nine months. X-ray of subtrochanteric osteotomy in surgery. Note cartilaginous defect in trochanteric area.

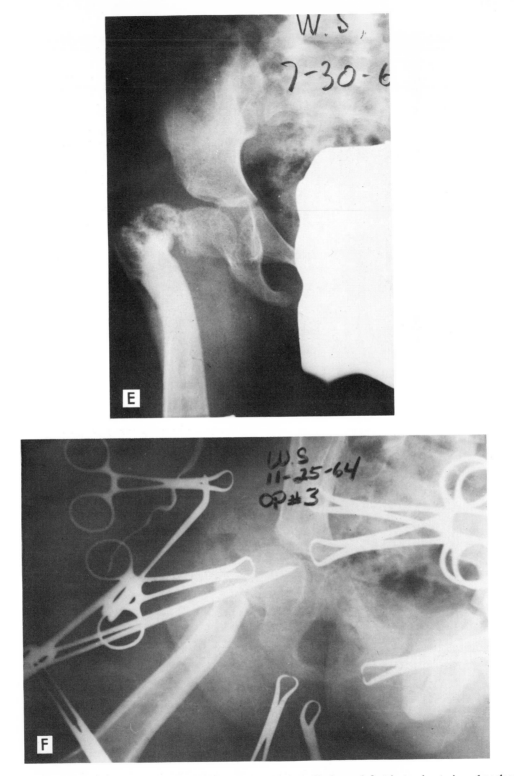

FIGURE 1-E   Same case at age five years, two months. Persistent varus with cartilaginous defect in trochanteric and neck portions
of femur.

FIGURE 1-F   Same case at age seven years, six months. X-ray at operation reveals bone continuity of shaft to femoral neck after excision
of cartilaginous defect.

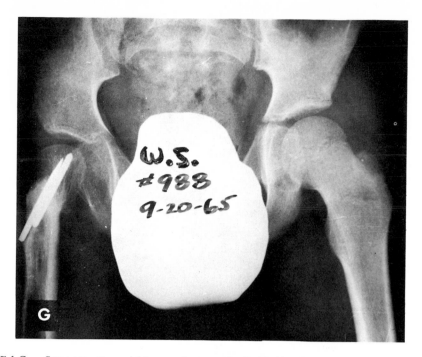

FIGURE 1-G   Same case at age eight years, four months. Stable hip with satisfactory shaft–neck angle.

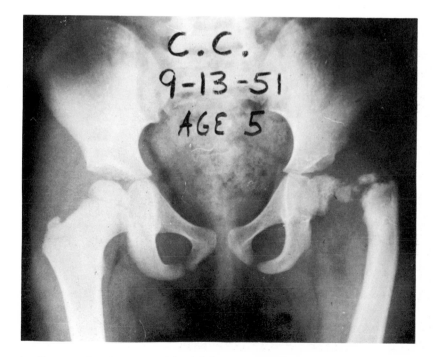

FIGURE 2-A   Age five years. Proximal femoral focal deficiency with cartilaginous defect in neck and trochanteric area.

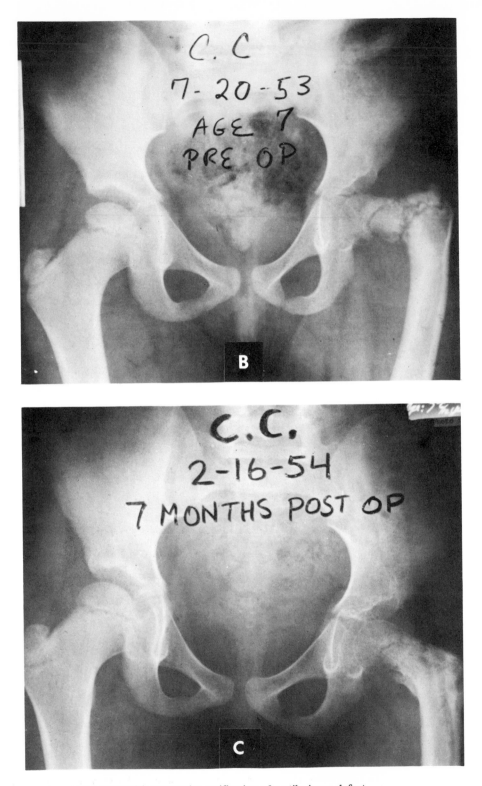

FIGURE 2-B   Same case at age seven years with progressive ossification of cartilaginous defect.
FIGURE 2-C   Same case at age eight years. Successful subtrochanteric osteotomy in presence of bone continuity of shaft and neck.

Contributors

GEORGE T. AITKEN, M.D., *Co-Medical Director*
Area Child Amputee Center, Division of Services to Crippled Children
Grand Rapids, Michigan

HARLAN C. AMSTUTZ, M.D.
The Hospital for Special Surgery, Cornell University Medical College
New York, New York

DIETRICH BOCHMANN, C.P.O. (C)
Prosthetic Service Department, Ontario Crippled Children's Centre
Toronto, Ontario, Canada

FINN O. GUNDERSON, Lt. Col., M.C.
Department of the Army
3rd Field Hospital, APO SF 96307

JOHN E. HALL, M.D., F.R.C.S. (C)
Chief, Amputee Clinic, Ontario Crippled Children's Centre
Chief, Division of Orthopaedic Surgery, Hospital for Sick Children
Toronto, Ontario, Canada

RICHARD E. KING, M.D.
Georgia Juvenile Amputee Clinic, Crippled Children's Service
P.O. Box 15089, Atlanta, Georgia

G. WILBUR WESTIN, M.D., *Chief Surgeon*
Shriners Hospitals for Crippled Children
Los Angeles, California